Fundamental Techniques in Veterinary Surgery

SECOND EDITION

CHARLES D. KNECHT, B.S., V.M.D., M.S.

Diplomate, American College of Veterinary Surgeons
Diplomate, American College of Veterinary Internal Medicine
Professor and Head, Department of Small Animal Surgery and Medicine
Auburn University

ALGERNON R. ALLEN, B.S., B.A., M.S.

Professor of Medical Art
Director of Medical Illustrations and Communications
School of Veterinary Medicine
Purdue University

DAVID J. WILLIAMS, A.A., B.A., M.A.

Associate Professor of Medical Art
Associate Director of Medical Illustrations and Communications
School of Veterinary Medicine
Purdue University

JERRY H. JOHNSON, D.V.M., M.S.

Diplomate, American College of Veterinary Surgeons
Practitioner, Lexington, Kentucky

W. B. SAUNDERS COMPANY
Philadelphia London Toronto Mexico City Rio de Janeiro Sydney Tokyo

W. B. Saunders Company: West Washington Square
Philadelphia, PA   19105

1 St. Anne's Road
Eastbourne, East Sussex BN21 3UN, England

1 Goldthorne Avenue
Toronto, Ontario M8Z 5T9, Canada

Apartado 26370 — Cedro 512
Mexico 4, D.F., Mexico

Rua Coronel Cabrita, 8
Sao Cristovao Caixa Postal 21176
Rio de Janeiro, Brazil

9 Waltham Street
Artarmon, N.S.W. 2064, Australia

Ichibancho, Central Bldg., 22-1 Ichibancho
Chiyoda-Ku, Tokyo 102, Japan

Library of Congress Cataloging in Publication Data

Main entry under title:

Fundamental techniques in veterinary surgery.

1. Veterinary surgery.   I. Knecht, Charles D. [DNLM:
   1. Veterinary medicine. SF911 F981]

SF911.F95 1980   636.089'7   80–52771

ISBN 0–7216–5463–0

Listed here is the latest translated edition of this book together
with the language of the translation and the publisher.

Spanish (*1st Edition*) — Editorial Acribia

Fundamental Techniques in Veterinary Surgery   ISBN   0-7216-5463-0

Last digit is the print number: 9   8   7   6   5

This book is dedicated to John R. Welser
who was a driving force for the first edition
and remains so for veterinary education.

PREFACE
to the Second Edition

The first edition of this text was treated well by the passage of time. Many were kind enough to send their compliments on the contents and many more to recommend it as a required text. To these and the others who invested their funds and attention to the text, we are indebted.

Others favored us with critical reviews. From these emerged a major change in content—the inclusion of techniques applicable to large domestic animals. The expertise of Jerry Johnson was solicited and will be recognized in this edition. Two of our previous authors have gone on to more challenging and time-consuming positions.

We particularly miss the talents of John Welser, for it was he, more than anyone, who made the first edition a reality. John suggested the project, helped organize the text, read every word, and supported our efforts. As dean of Michigan State University School of Veterinary Medicine, his time spent in administration does not permit participation in this edition. Therefore, this edition is dedicated to Dr. Welser in recognition of his primary efforts and continued support.

Our thanks are due the excellent staff at W. B. Saunders, the support provided at Purdue University, Auburn University, and the University of Missouri, and the students who continually advance the need for newer information.

PREFACE
to the First Edition

Surgery is a combination of both science and art. A good surgeon should have a firm foundation in and a working knowledge of anatomy, physiology, pathology, and diagnostic medicine. The early years of medical training are devoted to the acquisition of this knowledge.

At the appropriate time the medical student is expected to apply his or her knowledge to medical and surgical treatment. Regrettably, the beginning surgeon may lack expertise and thus cause harm by carelessly or ill-advisedly applying his or her techniques and skills. Not every medical student will become a skilled surgeon, but each should be capable of doing more good than harm to the patient. The fundamental skills can be learned by means of demonstrations, films, and models; the art of application will require experience.

This text is designed to present the fundamental surgical techniques in a usable form for the medical student. Although written essentially for the veterinary surgeon, it is applicable to any medical or paramedical student. It is not a short course in techniques; the technical procedures described here are used as examples of application only. Nor is it a work to be used in place of basic knowledge of the structures and function of animals; such use would be a disservice to all. Our hope is that it will provide a seedbed of technical knowledge from which the art of surgery may bloom.

The authors have diverse skills and interests. The balance of participating surgeons, teachers, and illustrative communicators was carefully chosen to provide all involved with the best possible format for sharing with each other and the reader both the science and the art of surgery. The senior author is indebted to each coauthor for his talents, diligence, and enthusiasm.

We are all indebted to many persons for technical support: to Thomas Wilson for assistance in the photographic procedures and embellishments; to Miss Deborah Goldsmith for her stenographic skills and untiring good humor; to Mr. George Laurie, of W. B. Saunders, for his technical advice and skill; and to Jean Knecht for indexing.

We are further indebted to Mr. Carroll Cann of W. B. Saunders and Dr. John Oliver of Purdue for their support in this venture. Most of all, we must thank our wives for their patience, understanding, and support during the years. We thank our students as well for expressing the need for such a work and for critically reviewing the results of our efforts.

CONTENTS

Chapter 3
SUTURE PATTERNS

Chapter 4
OPERATING ROOM CONDUCT

CONTENTS

Chapter 5
WOUND DRESSING

Chapter 6
WOUND DRESSINGS FOR THE HORSE

Chapter 7
APPLICATION OF TECHNIQUES

Chapter 8
CASTS AND SPLINTS FOR SMALL ANIMALS

1

SURGICAL INSTRUMENTATION

1

SURGICAL INSTRUMENTATION

The primary goal of the surgeon is the correction of disease states by physical intervention. This intervention, which may be by manipulation, incision, excision, or introduction of plastic repair, is, in itself, traumatic to the patient. The competent surgeon strives to minimize the damage that he himself must do to the patient.

The budding surgeon is presented with a plethora of tools that are, in the hands of others, the instruments of surgery. By increasing his knowledge and dexterity, the student should gain the ability to use the proper instrument at the proper time with minimal trauma to the patient.

CUTTING INSTRUMENTS

Scalpels

The scalpel is the primary cutting instrument of the surgeon. Early scalpels were simple blades shaped to a required configuration. The cutting edge dulled rapidly and, with repeated sharpening, became misshapen.

Scalpel handles with detachable blades were produced to eliminate the problems inherent with single piece scalpels. The prototype was the "Bard-Parker" spatula-like handle, which was produced in several sizes (Fig. 1–1). The handle was larger at the end opposite the blade and grooved to permit a stable grasp by the surgeon. In veterinary medicine, the number 3 and 4 handles are used in small and large animal surgery. Blades are available in various sizes and shapes (Fig. 1–1). The blades may additionally be ribbed along the non-cutting edge. This ribbing is applied to

stabilize the blade, but newer metals provide stability without such ribbing. A scalpel with the blade and handle packaged as a disposable unit is available.

The long, thin handle, which is more comfortable than the standard handle for some surgeons, is available for Bard-Parker blades. A small, rounded handle is also available with smaller disposable blades. The latter — Beaver blades — have gained popularity in ophthalmologic surgery and microprocedures.

The primary advantage of disposable blades for the surgeon and the patient is

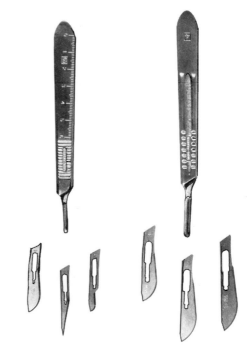

Figure 1–1 Bard-Parker scalpel handles and blades.

consistent sharpness. Most shapes and sizes are available in gas-sterilized packages; therefore, heat or chemical sterilization, either of which is a factor in dulling, is not necessary. It should be pointed out that a large selection of operating *knives* is still available. In veterinary surgery, these are most often used for special procedures (e.g., bovine teat surgery) or for non-surgical dissection in which minimal trauma is not essential (Fig. 1–2).

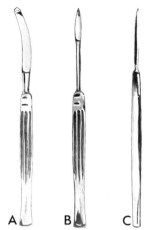

Figure 1–2 *A,* Teat bistoury; *B,* Tenotomy knife; *C,* Graefe knife.

The scalpel should be employed to cause minimal trauma to the tissues. The cutting surface should be *drawn across* the incision site to penetrate to the desired depth and *not driven in* the tissue like a wedge (Fig. 1–3). A single long stroke is more efficient, less traumatic to the tissues, and more likely to produce a smooth edge than are multiple small cuts. The longest possible blade surface should be in contact

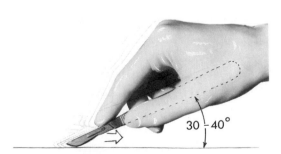

Figure 1–3 Cutting motion — #10 blade.

with the skin, rather than the shortest. As shown in Figure 1–3, the stroke with the number 10 blade should be made with the handle at a 30° to 40° angle from the line the cutting edge will follow. The thumb, middle, and ring fingers are used to grasp the handle, which rests in the palm of the hand. The index finger is placed on the upper edge of the cutting blade for stability; it should neither touch the skin nor obstruct the surgeon's view of his incision line. A pencil-grip of the scalpel should be used only when angling the blade would jeopardize surrounding tissue (Fig. 1–4).

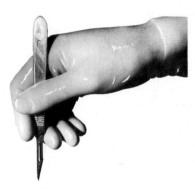

Figure 1–4 Pencil grip.

Electroscalpel

Electrosurgical currents are used to incise tissues or to coagulate small vessels. The result depends largely on the character and power of the sine or damped-sine wave produced. Most units (Fig. 1–5) may be adjusted to provide maximal incision or coagulation with minimal corollary function. In either, microcoagulation of tissue proteins results.

Most electrosurgical units provide a patient ground for return of current. The ground should cover a large surface area by contact with conductive paste or alcohol-soaked sponges. If a small return contact should occur, protein coagulation and tissue destruction will occur at the ground.

The surgeon using electroincision should minimize the contact area at the point of incision. A needle electrode is preferable to a blade for this purpose. Either should be held perpendicular to the tissues and moved rapidly through them.

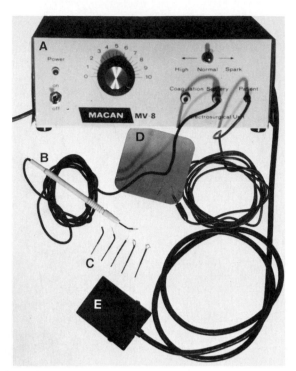

Figure 1-5 A Macan electrosurgical unit. A, Power unit; B, Handle; C, Electrodes; D, Grounding Plate; E, Foot Pedal.*

Only one tissue plane should be cut with a single pass. Skin and fascia are easily incised by electroincision. Fatty subcutaneous tissue is better incised with a cold scalpel or scissors. Muscle may be readily incised, but low frequencies should be avoided since these produce muscle contraction and result in irregular incisions.

Coagulation of small vessels may be performed with the coagulation mode and direct contact with the vessel end or contact with forceps grasping the vessel. A small ball electrode is generally used. Coagulation and heat increase the diameter of tissue destruction with prolonged application at a given site. The surgeon should utilize the minimal time necessary for coagulation. Vessels larger than 1 mm. in diameter should be ligated.

Some electrosurgical units provide a hand switch or capabilities for bipolar coagulation. In the latter, fine serrated forceps are incorporated in place of the electrode handle. The two tynes of the forceps are the

*Macan Engineering and Manufacturing Co., Chicago, Ill. 60622

active electrode and the passive electrode. Using this mode, a lesser amplitude of current is necessary for coagulation, and less surrounding tissue damage results.

Blood and balanced electrolyte solutions will disperse the electrode output in any mode. The tissues need not be dry, but adequate moisture control with moistened sponges, hemostats, and suction is essential to proper electrosurgical techniques.

Use of separate skin and deep blades is not necessary with electroincision because the electrode is sterilized by electrocoagulation during use.

In some instances, the electrode tip is held several mm. above the lesion, and a spark is allowed to gap. This technique (fulguration-desiccation) is used primarily for small benign growths. In veterinary medicine it has not been used extensively because of the desire to obtain specimens suitable for histopathologic examination of tissue type and adequacy of removal.

Heat and Cold

Because of the severe and extensive damage to surrounding tissues, incision by burning is never recommended. Incision with instruments generating temperatures below freezing (cryoincision) is being investigated.

Cryosurgery

Cryosurgery has been used extensively in the last five years for the removal of small to large masses that might otherwise require tedious and time-consuming dissection. Small skin growths, acral dermatitis, perianal adenomas, oral and nasal neoplasms, and perianal fistulae have been treated with cryoexcision with variable results.

Since protein coagulation and cell destruction result from freezing, the problem of immediate hemorrhage is avoided. Later hemorrhage associated with the tissue slough seven to 10 days after cryosurgery has been observed. Cicatrization has also been observed in the perianal area. Isolated reports of vascular emboli have been reported from use in the nasal cavity, which is a potentially serious complication when cryosurgery is used in or near cancellous bone.

A variety of cryosurgical instruments are available (Fig. 1–6). A proper instrument should permit a rapid freeze and slow thaw (usually done twice) and adequate monitoring of the depth of the freeze in degrees at the desired tissue level by thermoreceptors.

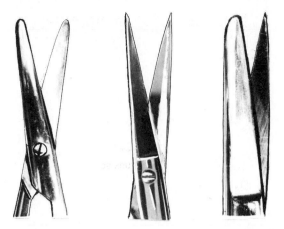

Figure 1–7 Point types (left to right): blunt-blunt, sharp-sharp, and sharp-blunt.

(straight or curved), and by the type of cutting edge (plain or serrated). The style depends upon the wishes of the designer and the surgeon. For most operative procedures, either Mayo or Metzenbaum scissors (Figs. 1–8 and 1–9) are excellent, although the latter style is thin and of limited use for dissection of dense tissues. Sistrunk dissecting scissors are preferred by some surgeons (Fig. 1–10).

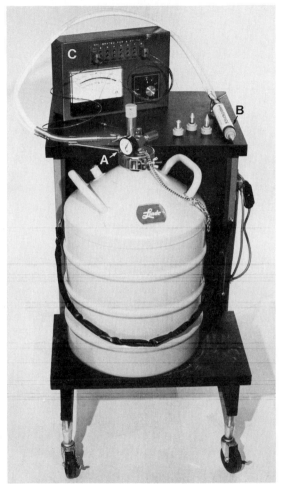

Figure 1–6 Union Carbide cryosurgery unit. *A,* Nitrogen source with regulator; *B,* Probe; *C,* Thermosensor with probes.*

Scissors

Operating scissors are available in various lengths, shapes, and weights. They are generally classified by the type of points (blunt-blunt, sharp-sharp, sharp-blunt, as in Fig. 1–7), by the shape of the blades

---

*Linde Cryogenic Equipment, Union Carbide Corporation, Speedway, Ind. 46224

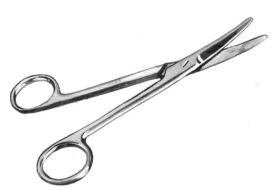

Figure 1–8 Mayo scissors.

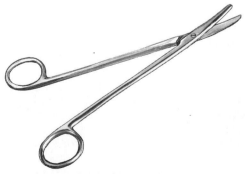

Figure 1–9 Metzenbaum scissors.

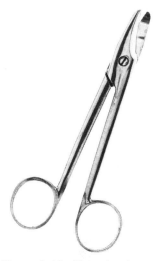

Figure 1–10   Sistrunk scissors.

Although some workers have discouraged the use of scissors for general incision of tissue planes, proper use will lessen the trauma inherent in a scissor cut. The procedures to follow in cutting with scissors are fairly straightforward:

The surgeon *must* press the handles of the scissors together, engaging the blades (Fig. 1–11). This is a natural action for the right-handed surgeon but requires considerable effort and practice on the part of the left-handed surgeon.

The surgeon *must* hold the scissors with the ring finger and thumb inserted in

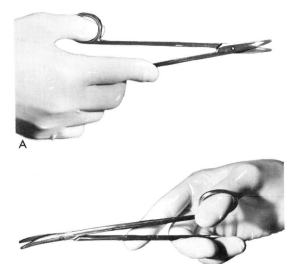

Figure 1–11   Grip for holding scissors.

the ring of the scissors, with the index finger guiding the scissors by its placement on the shaft. The finger or thumb must not be allowed to "fall through" the handle; the scissors rings should not rest close to the end of the first phalanx — rather, they should be kept near the last joint of the finger.

The surgeon *must* hold the scissors steady until the tissue or suture is severed. Many student surgeons withdraw the scissors while cutting. This practice may be likened to an action one finds in football: a receiver will take his eye off the pass to run for the end zone — and then drop the ball. Scissors do not cut well while being withdrawn.

The surgeon *must* use the end of the blade for cutting tissues, but he should *not* completely close the scissors if the incision is to be continued. A series of short cuts, made by closing the scissors at each bite, will result in a ragged incision. The scissors may be nearly closed, advanced, and closed again. A preferred technique is to (1) insert one blade below the tissue plane, (2) partially close the blades, and (3) press the scissors forward to cut the tissue in one continuous motion (Fig. 1–12).

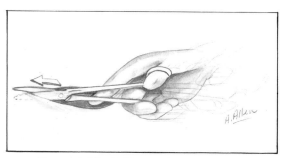

Figure 1–12   Cutting motion — scissors.

Scissors may also be used for blunt separation of tissue by inserting the points and *opening* the handles. Muscles and fat may be easily separated by this technique, but it should never be used for dense tissues (fascia, peritoneum, skin).

Suture scissors should be used to cut suture material (Fig. 1–13). Operating scissors should not be used for sutures. Most suture scissors are short and heavy and have serrated blades. The design permits use on heavy suture material or wire. In the in-are lighter in weight and have a sharp, thin point for introduction below the suture (Fig. 1–15). The cutting surface of one blade is hollowed out to prevent the suture from being lifted excessively during suture removal.

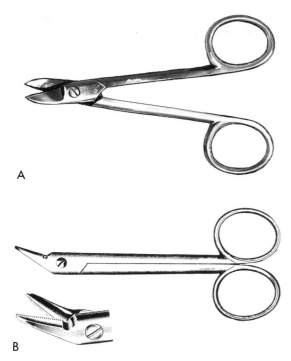

Figure 1–13   Suture scissors.

terest of economy, some veterinary surgeons cut sutures with the base of their operating scissors. This procedure appears to be an example of false economy. Suture scissors should be held in one hand with the palm up. The index finger of the opposite hand may be used to stabilize the blade (Fig. 1–14).

Suture scissors should not be confused with scissors for suture removal. The latter

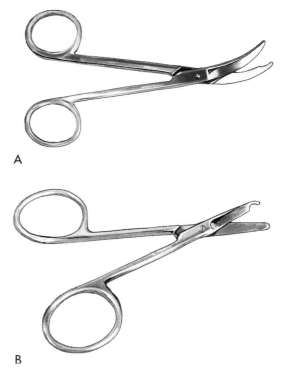

Figure 1–15   Spencer suture removal scissors.

Bandage scissors are equipped with a flattened, blunt tip on the lower blade (Fig. 1–16). This tip is introduced under the bandage without endangering the skin.

Cast cutting scissors and shears are useful for cutting thin layers of plaster (Fig. 1–17). Thicker plaster should be cut with an oscillating cast cutter (see Fig. 8–69).

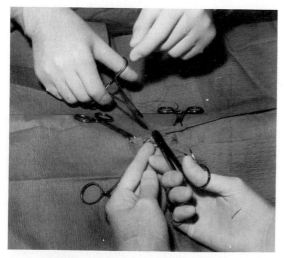

Figure 1–14   Use of suture scissors.

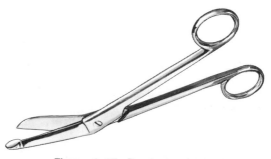

Figure 1–16   Bandage scissors.

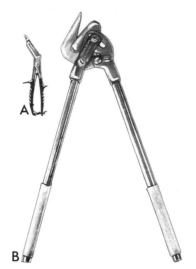

Figure 1–17 *A,* Cast cutting scissors; *B,* Cast cutting shears.

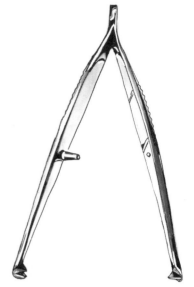

Figure 1–19 Rat tooth forceps.

FORCEPS

Forceps vary in both shape and use. The following classification is based upon use.

Dressing and Tissue Forceps

Dressing and tissue forceps consist of two tines or blades that are connected much like a wishbone and are designed to spring open (Fig. 1–18). The sides of the blades are wide and grooved in the middle for ease of handling with the thumb and forefingers.

The grasping surfaces (tips) may be smooth or may have teeth. Tissue forceps with large teeth should be used sparingly and only on the skin and more dense tissues (Fig. 1–19). Smooth-tipped tissue dressing forceps are recommended for handling other tissue planes and viscera, including blood vessels. A compromise is found in the Adson forceps (or in similar forceps), which have very small teeth on each edge of the tips (Fig. 1–20). These fine teeth cause minimal trauma, and the forceps as a whole stabilize tissue with minimal pressure. In addition, the Adson tissue forceps have a wider blade for thumb and finger pressure.

Russian thumb forceps have been advocated for use on soft tissues but lack the wide blade for ease of handling (Fig. 1–21). In operative practice, the forceps should not be held in the palm of the hand; rather, they should be held in the same manner as one would hold a pencil (Fig. 1–22). The forceps should be held in the lesser hand — that is, in the left hand of the right-handed surgeon and in the right hand of the left-handed surgeon.

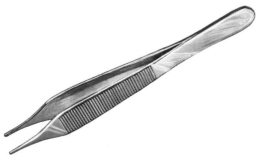

Figure 1–18 Ewald tissue forceps.

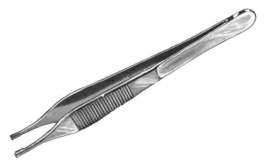

Figure 1–20 Brown-Adson tissue forceps.

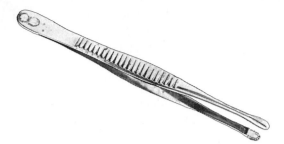

Figure 1–21 Russian thumb forceps.

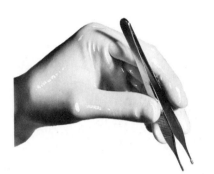

Figure 1–22 Holding the tissue forceps.

Hemostats

Hemostatic forceps are used to clamp and hold vessels. They vary from 3″ mosquito forceps to 9″ angiotribes. Each is equipped with a box lock so that it may be applied and left in position. Most hemostatic forceps have transverse grooves on the inside surface of the tips. The grooves may cover a portion or all of the tips. A variety of groove patterns are available and serve the surgeon well if used properly.

Rochester-Pean forceps are transversely grooved throughout the length of the tips and are useful for the control of large tissue bundles and vessels (Fig. 1–23). The

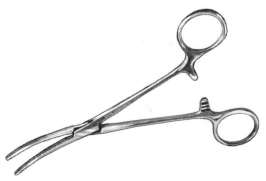

Figure 1–23 Rochester-Pean forceps.

Ochsner modification has large teeth located at the tip ends that prevent slippage of the forceps in the tissues (Fig. 1–24). Unfortunately, the teeth are generally an inconvenience. Rochester-Carmalt forceps have longitudinal grooves with cross grooves at the ends of the tips (Fig. 1–25). This modifi-

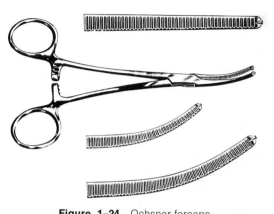

Figure 1–24 Ochsner forceps.

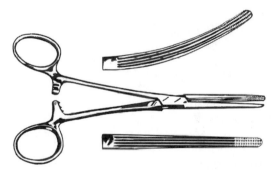

Figure 1–25 Rochester-Carmalt forceps.

cation is particularly useful because it facilitates removal of the hemostat during ligation. Kelly forceps are transversely grooved on the distal half of the tips only and should be used for small vessels (Fig. 1–26). Mosquito forceps are designed for use on small bleeders (Fig. 1–27).

The following guidelines for the proper use of hemostatic forceps should be kept in mind:

1. Use the smallest forceps that will accomplish the needed hemostasis.
2. Grasp only as much tissue as necessary.
3. Use the tip of the forceps rather than the middle or base.
4. Apply mosquito forceps to small

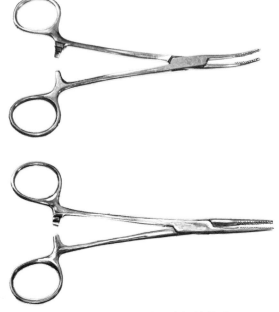

Figure 1–26   Curved and straight Kelly forceps.

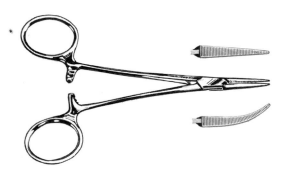

Figure 1–27   Halsted mosquito forceps.

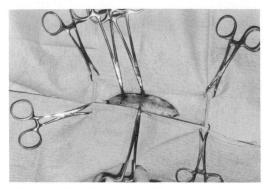

Figure 1–28   Hemostasis with mosquito forceps.

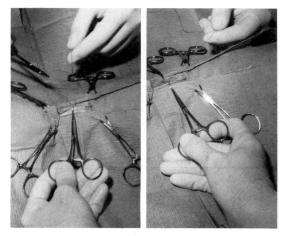

Figure 1–29   Removal of mosquito forceps.

bleeders perpendicular to the surface.

5. Apply other forceps perpendicular to the vessel to be ligated, compressing the widest dimension of the stump.

6. Apply mosquito forceps to surface bleeders so that they fall lateral to the incision with the concave part of the curve down (Fig. 1–28). In deeper locations, such as the abdominal cavity, place the forceps with the concave side up.

Hemostats may be removed by holding one finger loop between the thumb and finger and lifting the opposite finger loop (Fig. 1–29). Whether this technique is done right- or left-handed, the finger and thumb are not placed in the holes of the forceps.

Other Forceps

Other forceps differ in the shape of the tips. *Allis* tissue forceps are designed to provide minimal tissue trauma with maximal holding power (Fig. 1–30). The area of tissue contact is small but is perpendicular to the direction of pull. *Babcock* tissue forceps are similarly designed. Neither should be used to grasp and hold viscera, because

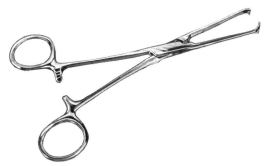

Figure 1–30   Allis tissue forceps.

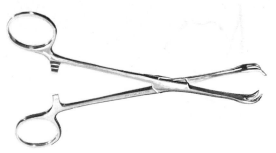

Figure 1–31 Vulsellum forceps.

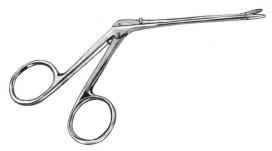

Figure 1–33 Alligator forceps.

tissue trauma can result. Vulsellum forceps have fenestrated jaws for a firm grasp of tissues but produce considerable trauma (Fig. 1–31). Duval and Lovelace lung-grasping forceps have tips shaped like triangles, with the base at the end (Fig. 1–32); they are pliable to prevent trauma to the lung.

Two other types of forceps commonly used in veterinary surgery are alligator and serrefine forceps. Alligator forceps have jaws at the end of the tips that open and close by movement of a long sliding shaft attached to standard but offset handles (Fig. 1–33). The unique structure permits introduction and grasping through a narrow opening; this procedure is not possible with forceps that open at a central pivot point.

Alligator forceps are available with serrated or rat tooth tips.

Serrefine forceps (bulldog clamps) are spring forceps resembling thumb forceps, with the exception that serrefine blades cross (Fig. 1–34). The spring closes the serrated, slightly hourglass-shaped tips;

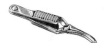

Figure 1–34 Serrefine forceps.

digital pressure is needed to open, rather than close, the forceps. The tips are flat on the inner serrated surface and convex on the outer. Serrefine forceps are used to temporarily occlude blood flow in medium-sized vessels. Serrefine forceps are particularly useful for hemostasis during nephrotomy.

Hemoclips

Several forms of metal clips are available for the ligation of small vessels (Fig. 1–35). The clips, which are bent pieces of

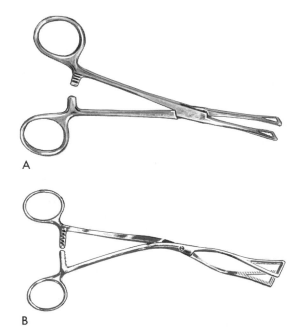

A

B

Figure 1–32 *A*, Duval lung-grasping forceps; *B*, Lovelace lung-grasping forceps.

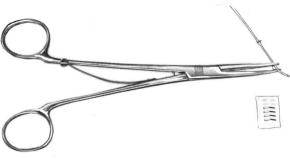

Figure 1–35 Hemoclips*

*Versa Clip — Pitman Moore Co., Washington Crossing, N.J. 08560.

metal (silver or steel, for example), are picked from a storage cartridge and are applied with special forceps. Some clips close from the bent to the open end; others are designed to close at the open end first. Hemoclips ars most useful for deep vessels where ligatures are difficult to apply.

NEEDLE HOLDERS

Most needle holding forceps resemble hemostatic forceps with these exceptions: Needle holding tips are shorter and heavier and are grooved in a cross pattern. In addition, many needle holders have a longitudinal groove in the tip to assist in grasping the needle.

Needle holders may be long (Mayo-Hegar, Metzenbaum — Fig. 1–36) or short (Derf — Fig. 1–37). They may have curved or angled tips (Metzenbaum, Finochietto). Although most needle holders have finger holes in the handles, some resemble pliers (e.g., Crile-Mathiew needle holders) or are spring forceps closed by thumb pressure against a lever (Kalt, Castroviejo). The Kalt needle holder requires release of a thumb catch to free the needle. Mathiew and Boynton forceps have an open box lock that is

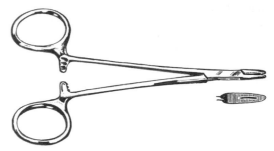

Figure 1–37 Derf needle holders.

released by pressing the lock past the point of maximum closure.

A fairly common technique for handling needle holders involves removal of the finger and thumb from the finger holes to grasp the shaft of the forceps loosely. The finger and thumb are replaced in the finger holes when it becomes necessary for the surgeon to grasp the needle and tie the suture. This procedure, in which suturing is a combination of grasping and releasing the needle holders, is *not* recommended (unless holders without finger holes are used). The beginning surgeon should place the thumb and ring finger in the finger holes and *should not* remove them. Time will not be lost grasping and releasing the forceps and, with a bit of practice, a totally satisfactory suture technique can be mastered. The index finger of the hand grasping the needle holders is used to direct them (as is done with hemostatic forceps).

A combination scissors and needle holder is available in several forms (Olson-Hegar, Gillies). The combination instrument has a needle-holding jaw on the tips of the scissors blades (Fig. 1–38). The instrument is useful for the closure of skin and other superficial layers. It should not be used for deep suturing or dissection because of the placement of the blades and the likelihood of accidentally severing sutures.

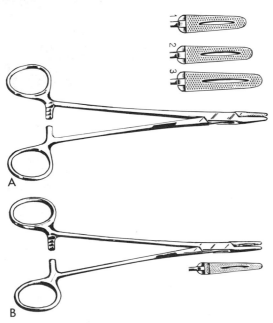

Figure 1–36 *A*, Mayo-Hegar néédle holders; *B*, Metzenbaum needle holders.

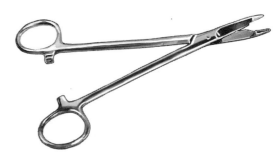

Figure 1–38 Olson-Hegar scissors/needle holder.

A unique instrument for suturing combines a stationary needle and a bobbin for holding suture material. The prototype is the Singer surgical sewing machine; the commonly used instrument today is the Suturator (Fig. 1–39). The design includes:

1. a bobbin placed in an enclosed handle;

2. a spring-mounted hold on the bobbin that may be released by thumb pressure on a button;

3. an opening for passage of the suture material from the bobbin to the needle;

4. a needle that can be locked by a thumb screw; and

5. two holes in the shaft of the needle that are large enough for passage of the suture material.

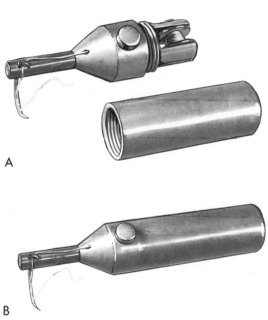

A

B

Figure 1–39 Suturator.

The bobbin is loaded with a suitable suture material, and the instrument is autoclaved. In use (Fig. 1–40), the needle is introduced through the tissue plane from one side of the incision through the other. The suture material is grasped and pulled as the bobbin is released to roll freely. When sufficient suture material is delivered, the needle is withdrawn, the bobbin button is released to fix the suture, and a one-hand knot is tied. The suture is then cut with

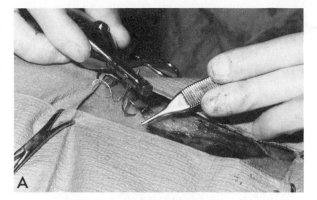

A

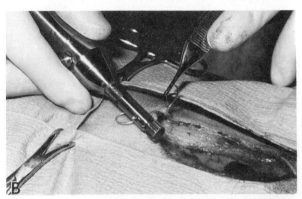

B

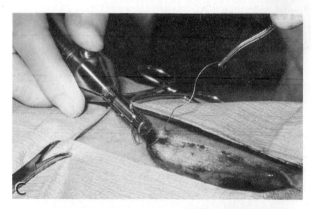

C

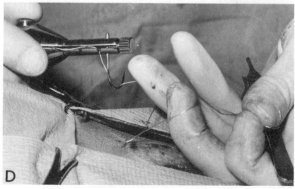

D

Figure 1–40 Use of the suturator.

scissors or, in certain instances, the needle edge. The instrument is useful and allows rapid suturing, but it limits the range of suture materials that can be used. In addition, it must be steam or gas sterilized.

The student surgeon is often heard to remark on the difficulty of "pushing the needle" through the skin. Attention to four procedural items will help:

1. Use the correct needle for the tissue (tapered needles do not pass readily through the skin).

2. Grasp the tissue with thumb forceps as close to the point of entrance of the needle as possible to immobilize the skin.

3. Grasp the needle at the bottom of the curve rather than near the eye; this allows a straighter pass through the skin.

4. Place the skin over the needle; don't push the needle through the skin.

RETRACTORS

Retractors are used to facilitate exposure of the surgical field with as little trauma as possible; they may be hand-held or self-retaining.

Hand-held retractors are bands of stainless steel with the ends bent to hold tissues or to be held in the hand (Figs. 1–41 and 1–42). The ends may be hooked, curved, toothed, or spatula-shaped. They are an invaluable aid to the surgeon, but their use requires active participation by an assistant.

Self-retaining retractors are held open by a box lock, spring, or worm gear. Box lock and spring retractors are used in incisions under minimal compressive forces. The most frequently used of these retractors are the Gelpi muscle retractors (Fig. 1–43) and the Weitlaner mastoid retractors (Fig. 1–44). Larger retractors are available for deep

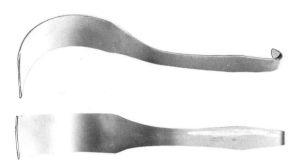

Figure 1–42   Devan retractor.

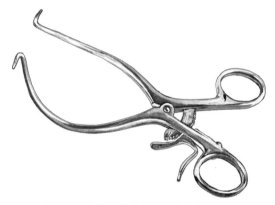

Figure 1–43   Gelpi muscle retractor.

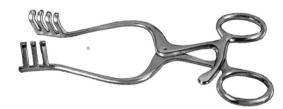

Figure 1–44   Weitlaner mastoid retractor.

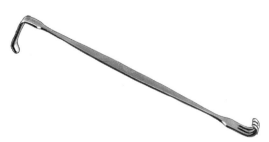

Figure 1–41   Senn retractor.

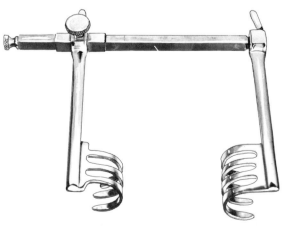

Figure 1–45   Frazier retractor.

cervical and lateral lumbar retraction (Figs. 1–45 and 1–46). The Balfour retractor provides three-point fixation and is useful in retraction of the abdominal musculature (Fig. 1–47). For rib retraction, a stronger retractor is required; it should have blunt tips and provide a mechanical advantage for the surgeon. The *Finochietto* retractor is useful in thoracotomies in the dog.

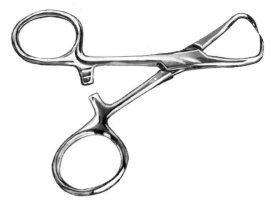

Figure 1–48 Plain Backhaus towel clamp.

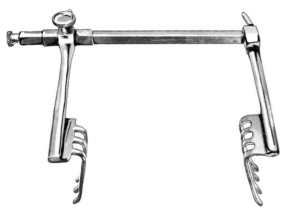

Figure 1–46 Temple-Fay retractor.

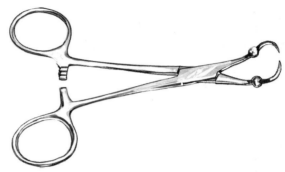

Figure 1–49 Backhaus towel clamp with ball stop.

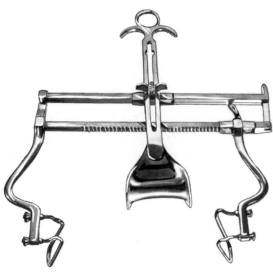

Figure 1–47 Balfour retractor.

TOWEL CLIPS

Towel clips are forceps with pointed tips that curve and joint like ice tongs to hold drapes and towels in position on the skin (Fig. 1–48). They are available with a metal bead on each tip that prevents the drape from advancing up the tips (Fig. 1–49). Small (3″) Backhaus towel clips are preferred for small animal surgery, but larger clips are often used on large animals.

Towel clips should be placed at a 45° angle to the incision at the four corners of the draped area. Clips should be secured to a minimal amount of skin through the covering drapes, which overlap at 90° angles (as in Figs. 1–28 and 1–40).

Draping the Patient

In general, contamination is less likely to occur with disposable drapes than with cloth drapes. In any event, more contamination results from faulty draping technique than from a specific type of drape.

If cloth drapes are used, they should be double layer or of suitable impervious material. The drape should not be plastic or rubber because of the danger of overheating the patient.

Fenestrated drapes are commonly used in veterinary surgery for routine elective surgical procedures such as ovariohysterec-

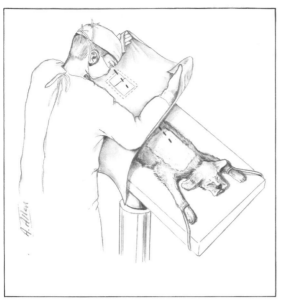

Figure 1–50   Fenestrated draping.

tomy, castration, and onychectomy. Such drapes are acceptable if the fenestration is the correct size and the drape is sufficiently large. The fenestration should almost exactly equal the incision area. Smaller drapes are not appropriate for small dogs; the surgeon should remember he is covering the table, not just the animal.

The fenestrated drape generally should be unfolded before application. It is held with the long axis of the fenestration parallel to the proposed incision. The surgeon must look through the opening to apply the drape (Fig. 1–50). Larger drapes may be folded above the fenestration with the folds toward the surgeon. The drape may then be applied and unfolded in a single motion without contamination.

Four corner drapes are applied one by one in a clockwise or counterclockwise direction (Fig. 1–51). Each drape should be

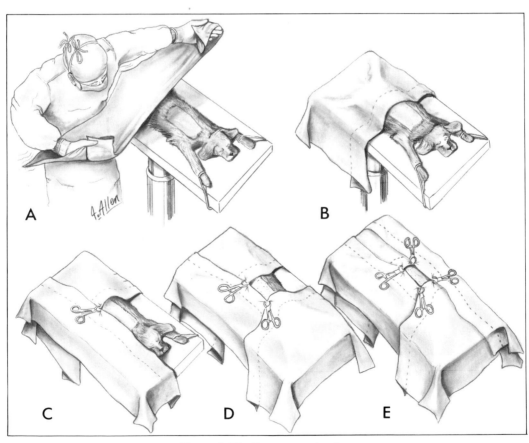

Figure 1–51   Four corner draping.

unfolded, and a 6″ to 8″ edge should be folded under, i.e., toward the patient. Each drape should then be "flown" to the point of final application. *Neither fenestrated nor regular drapes should be dragged to the incision site.* Only minor drape adjustment may be made without contaminating the underside of the drape and carrying the contamination to the incision area. The first drape is applied without contaminating the surgeon's gown on the undraped table. It should be applied in a position that will not be altered by gravity. The second drape is applied at a 90° angle to the first and a towel clip is applied. The process is then repeated around the incision. One drape should extend from the instrument table to the incision site to prevent contamination from the bottom of the instrument tray.

Accessory Draping

Several procedures in addition to normal draping are used to lessen contamination from the skin. *Towelling-in* is the term used to indicate that accessory drapes are attached to the skin to cover the skin between the existing drapes (Fig. 1–52).

The towelling shown in Figure 1–52 is placed around an incision made through the skin and subcutaneous tissue. A towel with one edge folded under (as is seen in regular drapes for application) is placed at the perimeter of the incision (Fig. 1–52A). A second towel is applied to cover both the first towel and the incision. Towel clips are applied to the skin through the unfolded towel, which is then drawn back to cover the clips (Fig. 1–52B, C). The first towel is unfolded to cover the incision (Fig. 1–52C), and towel clips are applied before the towel is folded back (Fig. 1–52D). Additional clips may be placed at each end to keep the towels from separating (Fig. 1–52E).

Proper draping of the limb is essential for good orthopedic surgery (Fig. 1–53). The limb is suspended by adhesive tape or a towel clamp clipped to tape on the foot during clipping and scrubbing. A single drape is placed medial to the thigh and is clipped in position. A sterile adhesive plastic drape is used to grasp the foot as an assistant releases the clip or cuts the tape. The foot is fully enfolded in the plastic to cover all non-scrubbed surfaces. A double-layer stockinette, knotted at one end and rolled before sterilization, is placed over the plastic drape and the limb. The stockinette may be cut medially at the inguinal area and extended laterally over the hip. The stockinette-covered leg may then be low-

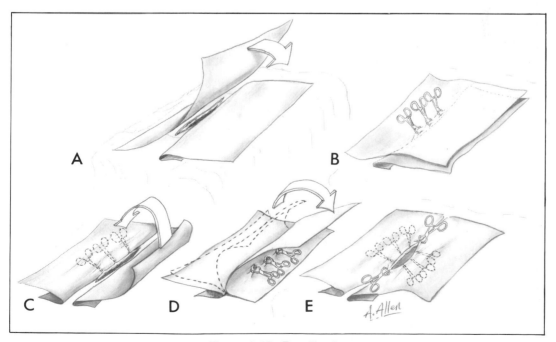

Figure 1–52 Towelling-in.

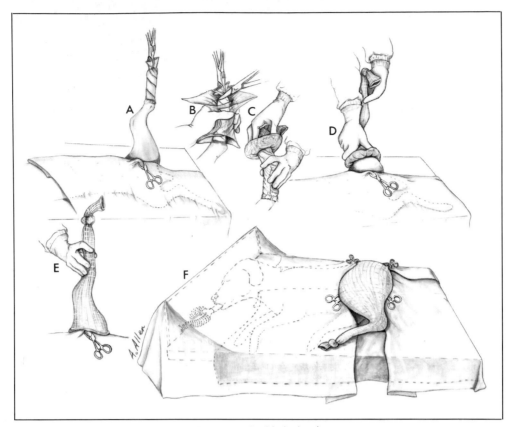

Figure 1–53 Limb draping.

ered to the positioned drape, and three other drapes should then be applied. Towel clamps join adjacent drapes and the stockinette to the skin.

At the proposed incision site, the stockinette is cut with scissors, and the skin and subcutaneous tissue are incised. The stockinette is then sutured to the subcutaneous tissue in a simple continuous inverting pattern on each side of the incision. These sutures will be removed before closure of the subcutaneous tissue.

Plastic drapes are available that are pre-glued or are applied to an adhesive sprayed on the skin. The incision is made through the drape. Such accessory drapes are beneficial if the edges do not loosen from the skin. Recent studies indicate that increased contamination at wound margins can occur if adherent drapes retract from the skin edges. Plastic drapes are useful in covering the non-scrubbed foot and the adhesive tape before application of the stockinette in orthopedic procedures.

Draping the Large Animal Patient

The large animal patient is draped for a ventral abdominal approach with an awareness that the entire animal and table must be draped. In Figure 1–54, a horse is positioned in dorsal recumbency following induction of general anesthesia. The hooves are cleaned of excessive debris. The lower limbs and hooves are covered with disposable rectal examination gloves. The surgical site is then clipped or shaved, and a thorough surgical scrub is applied. A sterile povidine-iodine pack may be placed and removed before final draping.

A modification of four-corner draping is used. The cranial abdomen, thorax, and forelimbs are covered with a single layer or several smaller overlapping drapes. Each rearlimb is similarly covered with a single drape, and a larger drape is used to cover the caudal abdomen, extending over the rearlimb drapes. Side drapes are applied and are clipped at the four corners of contact

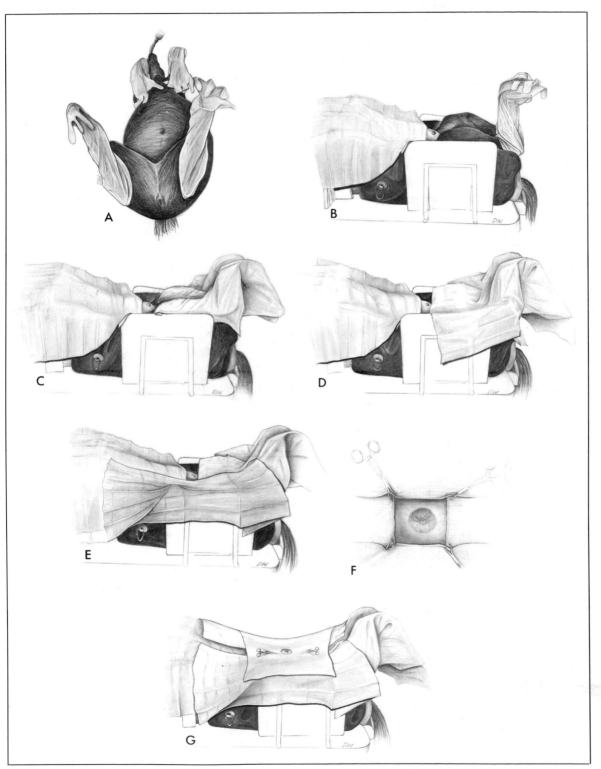

Figure 1–54 Draping for abdominal surgery in a horse.

with the cranial and caudal drapes with towel clamps. Finally, a fenestrated drape is applied over the four-corner drapes and is fixed in place with towel clamps placed cranially and caudally. The wound may be towelled-in after incision of the skin and subcutaneous tissue.

Draping for Standing Laparotomy

A standing laparotomy should be undertaken only on a cooperative patient on which a straightforward surgical procedure is planned. A clean, safe stock is necessary for restraint. The horse should be groomed, and the operative site should be clipped and scrubbed for aseptic surgery before the animal is put in the stocks.

A bleb of local anesthetic is deposited at the proposed sites of the towel clamps. A large sterile drape is applied to cover the horizontal bar of the stocks. Three-corner draping is then applied. An assistant should help draw the ends of the drapes to the opposite side as needed (Fig. 1–55).

The cranial drape is positioned slowly so as not to startle the horse and is attached to the mane with a hemostat. The next drape is placed over the back, and a towel clamp is applied where the first two drapes cross dorsal and cranial to the incision. A third, caudal drape is attached to the dorsal, horizontal drape dorsal and caudal to the incision site and to the cranial drape ventral to the incision site. When all drapes are applied, the exposed area is a triangle with the apex ventral to the incision. The skin and subcutaneous tissues should be towelled-in after incision.

In summary, draping is essential to good surgery. The following review might be helpful.

1. Drape the table in addition to the animal.

2. Drape between the operating and instrument tables.

3. Avoid contact with the operating table before it is draped.

4. Allow as little skin exposure as possible.

5. Take special care with orthopedic and neurosurgical procedures.

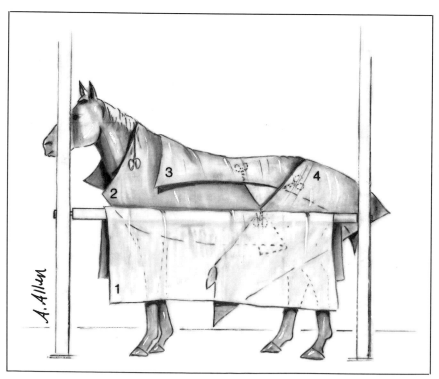

Figure 1–55 Draping for a standing laparotomy.

ORTHOPEDIC INSTRUMENTS

A complete discussion of orthopedic instruments is not within the scope of this book. However, a few basic types of instruments will be covered as examples of the equipment used in orthopedic surgery.

Rongeurs

Rongeurs are used to remove small particles of bone or to break larger particles (Figs. 1–56 and 1–57). Rongeurs are forceps with cupped, heavy tips that allow cutting of the bone. The cutting surfaces may be large or small. Rongeurs may be single or double action forceps; double action rongeurs increase the mechanical advantage for the surgeon, thus lessening the force needed to cut bone (Fig. 1–58).

Bone-cutting Forceps

Bone-cutting forceps are similar to rongeurs but have paired chisel-like tips for sharp cutting of bone (Fig. 1–59). They may be single or double action forceps.

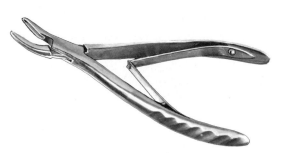

Figure 1–56 Rongeurs.

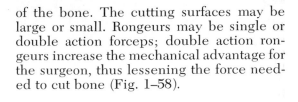

Figure 1–59 Bone-cutting forceps.

Trephines

Trephines are used to drill a cylinder of bone. They have T-handles and a cylindrical cutting blade. Some have central stylets for removing the bone from the shaft. The

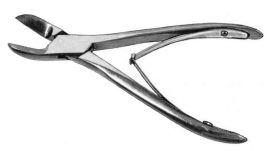

Figure 1–57 Alligator rongeurs.

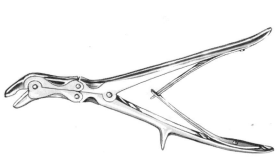

Figure 1–58 Stille-Luer double action duck-billed rongeurs.

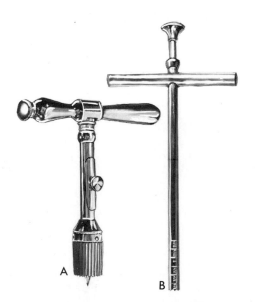

Figure 1–60 Trephines. *A,* Galt; *B,* Michel.

Michel trephine cuts only on the end of the shaft; the Galt trephine cuts bone on the end and on the outer perimeter of the trephine opening simultaneously (Fig. 1–60). A central trocar point facilitates introduction of the trephine; the trocar is removed after a circular trough is started in the bone. The Michel trephine lacks a trocar point; the bone may be roughened to facilitate introduction.

Other Cutting Instruments

Bone may also be cut with Gigli wire, a chisel, or an osteotome. The Gigli wire resembles closely packed barbed wire (Fig. 1–61) (the cutting wire is lined with densely packed wire ridges). Handles are available

for grasping the wire ends so that the wire may be sawed through the bone. Care should be taken to avoid overheating or otherwise injuring surrounding soft tissues with the Gigli wire.

A chisel may be used alone or with a mallet to shape or cut bone. The disadvantage of a chisel is that it tends to drift away from the beveled segment (Fig. 1–62). The osteotome is double-beveled and can be manipulated with minimal drift.

Bone-Holding Instruments

Bone-holding instruments may resemble forceps. They may be hand-held or self-retaining (Figs. 1–63 and 1–64). Kern and Verbrugge bone holders are available in small sizes (the names of which begin with the prefix "Baby"). Bone-holding forceps may be used to manipulate and hold fractured fragments and bone plates.

Bone clamps (e.g., Loman clamps) are available in large and small sizes for holding bones and plates (Fig. 1–65); they have

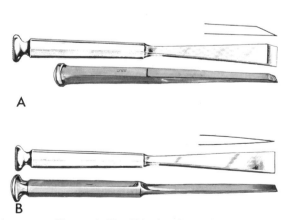

Figure 1–61 Gigli wire and handles.

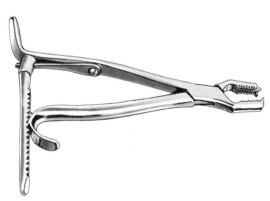

Figure 1–63 Kern self-retaining bone-holding forceps.

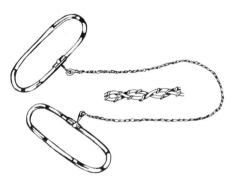

A

B

Figure 1–62 Chisel and osteotome.

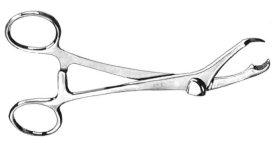

Figure 1–64 Verbrugge forceps.

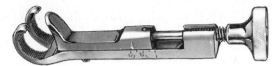

Figure 1–65 Loman bone-holding clamp.

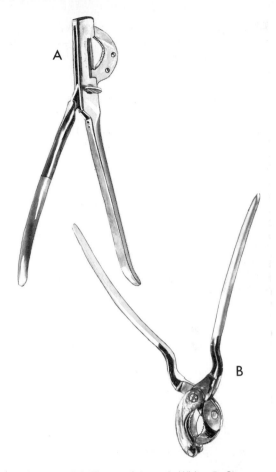

only limited use in manipulating bones. Bone may also be stabilized with stainless steel wire or steel bands (Parham band). The wire or band should be removed after appropriate fixation is applied.

Wire Twisters

Orthopedic wire may be applied by careful manipulation using two needle holders. A more consistent and reliable cerclage and hemicerclage may be obtained by the use of wire twisters (Fig. 1–66).

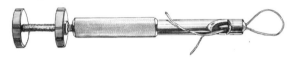

Figure 1–66 Bowen wire tightener.* The instrument severs the ends of the twisted wire.

Figure 1–67 Emasculators. *A,* White; *B,* Serra.

OTHER INSTRUMENTS

Numerous other routine and specialty instruments are available to the surgeon. Some are common to human and veterinary surgery. Others are common veterinary surgical instruments not used in humans. The White and Serra emasculators are used in the castration of large animals (Fig. 1–67).

A similar instrument used to grasp and amputate large appendages, i.e., in ovariectomy in the mare, is the ecrasier. A chain-ratchet ecraseur is shown in Figure 1–68.

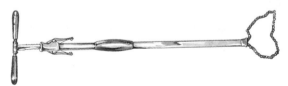

Figure 1–68 Chain ecraseur.

STANDARD SURGICAL PACKS

Institutional surgeons favor standard surgical packs for various types of proce-

dures. The type and number of instruments vary in the packs designed for general, orthopedic, neurosurgical, thoracic, ophthalmologic, or emergency use. Some surgeons prefer a standard basic pack with similar standardized specialty packs added for orthopedics, neurosurgery, and other disciplines. In either system, standardization of packs permits surgeons and technical staff to prepare for surgery with added efficien-

*Bowen and Co., Inc., Rockville, MD 20852

TABLE 1–1   Standard Surgical Packs

Items	Small Animals		Large Animals	
	General	Orthopedic	General	Orthopedic
Scalpel handles	2	2	2	2
Adson thumb forceps	1	1		
Thumb forceps (3 × 4 teeth)			1	1
Russian thumb forceps			1	
Mayo scissors		1	1	2
Metzenbaum scissors	1	1	1	1
Suture scissors	1	1	1	1
Mayo-Hager or Derf needle holders	1	1	2	2
Allis tissue forceps	4	4	8	8
Long Allis tissue forceps			4	4
Halstead mosquito forceps	8	10	4	4
Crile or Kelly forceps			12	12
Carmalt forceps	4			
Backhaus towel clamps	6	8	12	12
Grooved director	1			
Snook ovariohysterectomy hook	1			
Baby Kern or Lane bone-holding forceps		2		
Liston bone-cutting forceps		1		
Stille-Liston or Lempert rongeurs		1		1
Pituitary alligator rongeur				1
Kirschner hand chuck and key		1		
Pin and drill ruler		1		
Adson periosteal elevator		1		
Sayre periosteal elevator				1
Langenbeck periosteal elevator — broad				1
Langenbeck periosteal elevator — narrow				1
Senn retractor	2	2		2
Gelpi retractor		1		
Weitlaner retractor				1
Bone hook		1		
Bone curettes				3
Osteotomes				3
Bone mallet				1
Bandage scissors		1		
Saline bowl	1	1	1	1
Sponge forceps			1	1
Assorted needles in rack	1	1	1	1
Asepto syringe				1

cy. Standard packs are essential where two or more surgeons utilize the same equipment.

A standard general and orthopedic instrument list for small and large animals appears in Table 1–1. Supplementary instruments are added to fit the need of the specific procedure.

REFERENCES

Adams, R. and Fraser, R.: Plastic skin drapes. Am. J. Nurs., 1959, *59*:845–847.

Baker, J. and Braken, F. K.: Plastic fracture sleeve. Vet. Med., 1953, *48*:28.

Beck, W. C.: Justified faith in surgical drapes. Am. J. Surg., 1963, *105*:560–562.

Brinker, W. O.: Use of intramedullary pins in small animal fractures. N. Am. Vet., 1948, *29*:292.

Cahoon, J. R., and Paxton, H. W.: Metallurgical analyses of failed orthopedic implants. J. Biomed. Mater. Res., 1968, *2*:1.

Carney, J. P.: Rush intramedullary fixation of long bones as applied to veterinary surgery. Vet. Med., 1952, *47*:43.

Green, J. E., Hoerlein, B. F., Konde, W. N., and McBee, J. A.: The indications and limitations of the medullary nail in small animals. Corn. Vet., 1950, *49*:331.

Hall, D. E.: *Surgical Instrument Guide for Nurses.* Brooklyn, N.Y.: Ed. Weck & Co., 1954.

Jacobs, P. A. and Guten, G. N.: Compression fixations of bone. Wisconsin Med. J., 1967, *66*:412.

Veterinary Instruments. J. Sklar Mfg. Co., Long Island City, NY, 1978.

L'Esperance, F. A., Jr.: Clinical comparison of xenon-arc and laser photocoagulation of retinal lesions. Arch. Ophthalmol., 1966, 75:61.

Muller, M. E., Allgower, M., and Willenegger, H.: *Technique of Internal Fixation of Fractures.* New York: Springer-Verlag, 1965.

Ormrod, A. N.: Limb fractures in the dog and cat. J. Small Animal Prac., 1966, 7:155.

Partington, P. F.: Rubber bands as a replacement for rubber-shod clamps. Surg., 1970, 68:737.

Revie, R. W. and Greene, N. D.: Comparison of the in vivo and in vitro corrosion of 18-8 stainless steel and titanium. J. Biomed. Mater. Res., 1969, 3:465–470.

Weston, H. C.: The effect of age and illumination upon visual performance with close sight. Br. J. Ophthalmol., 1948, 32:645.

Veterinary Instruments. J. Sklar Mfg. Co., Inc., Long Island City, N.Y., 1978.

Yeager, M. E.: *Operating Room Manual.* New York: G. P. Putnam and Sons, 1965.

Zweng, H. C., Flocks, M., Kapany, N. S., Silbertrust, B. S., and Peppers, N. A.: Experimental laser photo-coagulation. Am. J. Ophthalmol., 1964, 58:353.

Note: Many of the instruments illustrated in this chapter are shown in the *Surgical Instrument Catalog* of the Lawton Company, Inc., 200 Anderson Ave., Moonachie, New Jersey 07074. The authors are indebted to the Lawton Company for permission to modify illustrations from their catalog for Figures 1–13, 1–24, 1–25, 1–27, 1–32, 1–36, 1–37, and 1–62.

2

SUTURE MATERIALS

2

SUTURE MATERIALS

HISTORY

The earliest methods of hemorrhage control were compression and immobilization of the wounded part. Application of mud, leaves, herbs, and poultices followed. Cautery in the form of a fire rod was used in ancient Egypt to control external hemorrhage. Hippocrates used cautery in the treatment of hemorrhoids and other diseases associated with bleeding.

Ligatures have been used for over 4000 years. Celsus, referring to the work of his predecessors, provided the first recorded description of the use of ligatures on vessels to control hemorrhage. In a comprehensive outline, he organized the treatment of hemorrhage into the application of pressure, styptics, astringents, ligatures, and, as a last resort, cautery. Galen, in the second century A.D., recommended silk for sutures. Arabian physicians used harp strings made from twisted and sun-dried sheep intestines.

Sutures and ligatures fell into disuse during the Dark Ages, when the hemostatic agents included boiling oil, boiling turpentine, molten lead, sulfur, and the hot iron. As the Renaissance began, Ambroise Paré (1510–1590) rediscovered ligatures, combining tight binding, mass compression, and ligation. In 1806, Dr. Phillip Physick produced sutures from kid and buckskin, but such absorbable sutures did not gain popularity until a century later. Joseph Lister introduced suture sterilization in 1869 as part of his work on asepsis. He also proposed that a clean, dry field be produced by elevation of the limb followed by application of a tourniquet. Later, Lister discovered that chromic acid impregnation of catgut delayed its absorption.

The tenaculum, a sharp hook with a wooden handle, was introduced before 1890. The tenaculum was used to grasp a bleeding vessel, and the handle was held in the surgeon's mouth while the vessel was tied. Twine, flax, and strips of cloth were used for ligation.

Other hemostatic agents introduced during the 1890s included bone wax, as advocated by Horsley, and gelatin, recommended by Carneb for local hemorrhage. In 1911, Cushing employed silver clips in neurologic surgery. In 1912, he collaborated with Bovie to produce an electrocautery unit for the control of hemorrhage in neurologic patients.

Stainless steel sutures were introduced in 1934, and synthetic sutures appeared in the 1940s. Development and improvement of suture materials continue and are noteworthy. Nevertheless, without the acceptance of Lister's antiseptic principles, the safe and widespread use of sutures and ligatures would not have been possible.

THE IDEAL SUTURE MATERIAL

The ideal suture material has not been found, although its characteristics have been known for at least a century. It should be nonreactive in the tissues, easy to handle, of monofilament composition, easy to completely sterilize, and should have high tensile strength in small sizes (8 pounds at size 4–0) in vivo and in vitro. It should maintain a knot without slippage, should absorb in a predictable manner in 30 to 60 days or until fragments are dissolved without harmful end products, and should be economical.

Since the ideal suture material does not exist, the surgeon must choose materials based on a knowledge of the attributes of that material and the conditions of the wound. If the normal strength of tissues, rate of recovery of strength after wounding, and the tensile strengths of sutures were known and predictable, selection would be simplified. Unfortunately, much information is either nonexistent or contradictory.

Recognizing that the ideal suture should be as strong as and not greatly stronger than the tissue being sutured, the surgeon faces a dilemma. In addition, biological reaction between suture materials and tissues can alter the mechanical properties of the suture and the healing process of the tissues. If biological processes reduce the suture strength (as occurs with catgut in a purulent wound), the suture size must be increased to compensate or another suture material must be chosen. The choice of material may be made to affect tissue reaction. Polyglycolic acid may be preferred in subcutaneous tissues because of the minimal tissue response and swelling that result. Catgut may be used as one of two layers in a diaphragmatic hernia repair to *increase* the inflammatory response.

Absorbable Sutures

Suture materials may be absorbable or nonabsorbable. The latter resist degradation, remaining in the tissues until removed. Absorbable sutures are digested and assimilated by the body during and after healing and may be of animal or synthetic origin. Animal collagen sources include gut, collagen, kangaroo tendon, and fascial strips.

Absorbable sutures are degraded primarily by macrophages as healing progresses. Collagen sutures are more rapidly absorbed in the presence of infection, increased blood supply, and naturally occurring enzymes, such as those found in the pancreas and small intestines. Certain absorbable sutures, such as polyglycolic acid, are hydrolyzed rather than absorbed. In either instance, the use of absorbable sutures should be questioned in infected or grossly contaminated wounds because they may be prematurely absorbed and may contribute to the suppurative process.

Surgical Gut

Surgical gut is derived from the submucosal layer of sheep or the serosa of cattle intestines, which is harvested, purified, and sterilized. The terms "catgut" (a derivative of kid gut, the intestine of a young lamb) and surgical gut are used synonymously. Surgical gut is classified by its degree of chromicization or tanning. Chromic suture is treated with chromic acid to lengthen and standardize absorption time and to reduce the intensity of soft tissue reaction to the gut.

The four types of surgical gut are:
Type A — Plain or untreated
Type B — Mild chromic treatment
Type C — Medium chromic treatment
Type D — Extra chromic treatment

Although the size of suture material may be defined by metric size (Table 2–1) or USP size (Table 2–2), the degree of chromicization and not the size determines the rate of absorption. Plain chromic treatment gut is absorbed within three to seven days, mild within 14 days, medium within 20 days, and extra within 40 days. The absorption rates are approximate and, as has been mentioned, depend on in vivo conditions. Standards for surgical gut are established in the U.S. Pharmacopeia. Catgut may be boilable (generally in 95 per cent alcohol, 0.5 per cent KHgI, and 5 per cent water), nonboilable (in zylol), or dry (treated with ethylene oxide or radiation). Glass tubes have been replaced with one plastic package sealed within a second and sterilized.

TABLE 2–1 U.S.P. Metric Gauge Sizes for Sutures

Metric Size (Gauge No.)	Limits on Diameter (mm)	
	Minimum	Maximum
0.01	0.001	0.009
0.1	0.010	0.019
0.2	0.020	0.029
0.3	0.030	0.039
0.4	0.040	0.049
0.5	0.050	0.069
0.7	0.070	0.099
1	0.100	0.149
1.5	0.150	0.199
2	0.200	0.249
3	0.300	0.339
3.5	0.350	0.399
4	0.400	0.499
5	0.500	0.599
6	0.600	0.699
7	0.700	0.799

TABLE 2–2 Comparable Size and Strength of Absorbable Sutures

USP Size	Metric Size (Gauge No.)			Limit on Knot-pull Strength (Kg.)*		
	Catgut	Collagen	Synthetic	Catgut	Collagen	Synthetic
10–0			0.2			
9–0		0.3	0.3		0.023	
8–0		0.5	0.4		0.045	
7–0	0.3	0.7	0.5	0.06	0.07	0.14
6–0	0.7	1	0.7	0.16	0.18	0.25
5–0	1	1.5	1	0.32	0.38	0.68
4–0	1.5	2	1.5	0.68	0.77	0.95
3–0	2	3	2	1.13	1.25	1.77
2–0	3	3.5	3	1.81	2.00	2.68
1–0	4	4	3.5	2.50	2.77	3.90
1	5	5	4	3.40	3.80	5.08
2	6	6	5	4.08	4.51	6.35
3	7	7	6	5.22	5.90	
4		8	6		7.00	

*Average of 10 strands tested.

Surgical gut is available in USP size 3, the heaviest, to 7–0, the thinnest. Specific size and tensile strength limits have been established (Table 2–2). The tensile strength is measured as knot strength rather than breaking force resulting from a straight pull because the strength decreases where knots are formed.

Surgical gut is tolerated by the tissues but does cause an inflammatory response. The liquids in which gut is packaged may be more irritating and should be rinsed from the gut before use. Surgical gut should not be allowed to remain submerged for long periods, however, because it is hydroscopic.

Surgical gut is easily handled and elastic, lessening the tendency to shrink and strangulate tissues. Because it is hydroscopic, knots tend to loosen. Three or more throws should be used in tying, and the ends should be cut slightly away from the knot to insure stability. Surgical gut is capillary and supports infection. It is, nevertheless, indicated for general ligation and for surgery of the gastrointestinal, urogenital, and parenchymatous organs. It is contraindicated for skin sutures and for implantation against nervous tissue.

Collagen

Collagen sutures are prepared from bovine tendon as homogeneous extrusion of collagen fibers. Collagen is uniform in size, ties well, and handles as well as catgut. It causes less inflammatory reaction than gut.

Although of good strength before use, it may be prematurely absorbed and may lose strength in vivo (Table 2–2).

Polyglycolic Acid

Polyglycolic Acid (P.G.A.) suture is woven from fine filamentous threads extracted from hydroxyacetic acid. Suture size is determined by the numbers of woven strands (Table 2–2). Polyglycolic acid sutures handle well, but the knots tend to slip. Two or more single throws covering a double throw are recommended. The suture also has a high coefficient of friction and tends to cut friable tissues. It is uniformly absorbed in 40 to 60 days.

The initial strength must be high because 25 to 33 per cent of the tensile strength is lost in vivo within seven days and 80 per cent is lost within two weeks. Polyglycolic acid remains stronger than catgut of comparable size for at least 15 days. It is, nevertheless, less reactive than surgical gut and has similar indications except it should not be used in tissues that heal slowly or in the mucosa of the urinary bladder or urethra. P.G.A. is prematurely absorbed in urine.

Polyglactic Acid

Polyglactin 910 (P.L.A.) is a synthetic absorbable suture that is a copolymer of lactide and glycolide. It is similar in use and attributes to P.G.A., except that it may be braided or monofilament. It maintains tensile strength for about three weeks and is absorbed within 90 days by hydrolysis.

Other Absorbable Suture Materials

Kangaroo tendon, fascia lata, and dura are other absorbable sutures. The first is taken from the tail of the kangaroo and is prepared similarly to surgical gut. It is stronger than catgut but has no other advantages and is rarely used.

Fascia lata and dura are prepared in strips for replacement and support in appropriate areas, but neither is commonly used.

Nonabsorbable Sutures

Nonabsorbable sutures are neither absorbed nor digested by the tissues, but many types fragment in time. Resisting degradation, they are encysted if buried in the tissues. Nonabsorbable sutures generally have high tensile strength and produce minimal tissue reaction. Multifilament sutures tend to support bacteria and cause more tissue reaction than monofilament sutures. The latter are more difficult to handle and are subject to slippage of knots.

Nonabsorbable sutures are grouped into metals, natural fibers, and synthetics. In addition, they may be treated to reduce capillarity (Type B) or non-treated (Type A). The U.S. Pharmacopeia divides nonabsorbable sutures into Classes I through III

(Table 2–3). Class I suture is silk or synthetic fiber suture that either has been twisted or braided or is monofilament. Class II sutures are composed of cotton or linen fibers or coated natural or synthetic fibers in which the coating adds thickness but not appreciable strength. Class III sutures are composed of monofilament or multifilament metal wire.

Metals

Gold, silver, copper, bronze, and tantalum have been utilized for suture materials. All except the last have been abandoned because of expense and a tendency to cause tissue reaction.

Tantalum is non-toxic, non-corrosive, physically and biologically inert, and is comparable in strength to wire. It tends to fragment when buried and is available in monofilament or multifilament forms.

Surgical stainless steel suture material was introduced in 1934 by Babcock. The 316L (low carbon) iron alloy is inert, non-corrosive, and will not support infection in vivo. Both monofilament and multifilament forms have high tensile strength, are easily sterilized, and are relatively inexpensive. The major disadvantage of wire is the difficulty in handling. Wire kinks easily, lacks elasticity, and is difficult to knot. The multifilament form is easier to handle but is more easily broken if kinked. Ends of either form should be tied, not twisted, and should

TABLE 2–3   Limits of Knot-pull Tensile Strength of Non-Absorbable Sutures

USP Size	Metric Size (Gauge No.)	Limits on Knot-pull Strength (Kg.)*			Comparable Wire Gauge
		Class I	Class II	Class III	
10–0	0.2	0.016	0.012	0.05	
9–0	0.3	0.036	0.024	0.06	
8–0	0.4	0.06	0.04	0.11	
7–0	0.5	0.11	0.06	0.16	
6–0	0.7	0.20	0.11	0.27	40
5–0	1	0.40	0.23	0.54	36
4–0	1.5	0.60	0.46	0.82	33
3–0	2	0.96	0.66	1.36	30
2–0	3	1.44	1.02	1.80	28
1–0	3.5	2.16	1.45	3.40	26
1	4	2.72	1.81	4.76	
2	5	3.52	2.54	5.90	24
3	6	4.88	3.68	9.11	18
4	6	4.88	3.68	9.11	18
5	7	6.16		11.4	
6	8	7.28		13.6	

*Average of 10 sterilized. The limits are 25 per cent higher for non-sterile Class I and Class II.

be cut close to the knot because the cut ends may irritate tissue. Neither should be pulled too tightly or tissues may be cut. Monofilament steel is satisfactory for use in infected wounds but multifilament steel is not. Swaged-on needles reduce the trauma caused by wire threaded through a needle.

Steel is appropriate for general closure, retention sutures, skin closure, and tendon repair. It is sold in Brown and Sharpe gauges 40 (the smallest) through 18 (the largest) or in U.S.P. diameter sizes 10–0 to 7 (Table 2–3, Class III).

Metal clips and **staples** are made of non-corrosive metals. Silver and stainless steel clips are used to ligate small vessels (Chapter 1), approximate wound edges, and secure accessory drapes to the edges of wounds.* Metal clips and staples are easy to apply and sterilize. They tend to increase scarring in skin unless removed early and require special equipment for application.

The Weck Instrument Company markets a metal clip that is applied to nonabsorbable sutures. Knots are supplanted by one metal clip on the suture on each side of the incision.†

Sutures of Natural Origin

Silk is the most widely used nonabsorbable suture material. It is prepared from threads spun by silkworm larvae. The strands are processed to remove natural waxes and gums, are twisted or braided, and are dyed to increase visibility. Braided suture is preferred because of its high tensile strength, ease of handling, and excellent knot stability. Silk is inexpensive, universally available, and readily sterilized. It is capillary unless treated with silicone or wax and should not be used in infected wounds. It retains tensile strength moderately well, losing 30 per cent in two weeks, nearly 60 per cent in one month, and nearly all in six to 12 months.

Silk is used in cardiovascular, ophthalmic, and gastrointestinal surgery and is an efficient suture provided that fine sizes are used, sterility is maintained, and it does not

protrude into the lumen of hollow organs, where it may form a nidus for calculi. Silk is available in sizes 9–0 to 5. Since silk loses strength in a fluid environment, it is packed dry.

Dermal suture is twisted silk fibers encased in a nonabsorbing coating of protein, such as gelatin. The coating prevents ingrowth of tissue cells and facilitates removal after skin closure. Dermal suture is particularly strong and is used primarily in plastic surgery.

Virgin silk suture is made from several natural silk fibers twisted to form a single strand of small diameter. Available in 8–0 and 9–0 sizes, virgin silk sutures may be closely applied with careful handling and form small knots. The nearly colorless material is temporarily dyed with methylene blue or iodine before use by some surgeons.

Cotton is made from long cotton fibers that are twisted into a strand. It is the weakest of the natural sutures but gains tensile strength when wet and should be moistened before use. Surgical cotton is well tolerated by the tissues, easy to use, easily sterilized, and knots well. Unfortunately, cotton is capillary and may contribute to the formation of sinuses and pustules. In addition, it sticks to wet surgical gloves, making it more difficult to handle.

Linen is twisted from long strands of flax. It is variable in diameter, lower in tensile strength than other nonabsorbable suture materials, and is rarely used.

Sutures of Synthetic Origin

Synthetic nonabsorbable sutures have found increased acceptance by veterinary surgeons. Many of the monofilament forms cause little tissue reaction, are noncapillary, and have high tensile strength. Some have a degree of plasticity, which promotes partial relief of tension to compensate for tissue swelling. Polymeric materials possess "memory," a built-in orientation produced by stretching during manufacture. The suture tends to straighten, and the knot may slip or untie. The combination of memory and a low coefficient of friction dictate that knots be carefully tied and contain more throws than knots with other suture materials. These characteristics are more marked with nylon and

---

*United States Surgical Corporation, New York, N.Y. 10022

†Suturematic Applier — Edward Weck and Company, Inc., a division of E.R. Squibb and Sons, Inc., Princeton, N.J. 08540

less with materials such as propylene, which has a small degree of plasticity.

Surgical **nylon** is a polyamide polymer that can be extruded into a non-capillary, monofilament strand or braided. Nylon produces minimal tissue reaction, has a high tensile strength, and is most often used for skin sutures. It degrades 15 per cent per year in tissues. Monofilament nylon has a low coefficient of friction and high memory. Four or more throws are needed for knot stability. Braided nylon handles easily and is stronger than silk. It is a multifilament strand, but it is generally treated to reduce capillarity.

Polymerized caprolactum is a twisted synthetic fiber suture with a smooth coating. It possesses high tensile strength and causes little tissue reaction. It is available in 0.3 mm (00), 0.4 mm (0), 0.6 mm, and 1.1 mm sizes in bulk rolls and in spools soaked in antimicrobial fluid. Use of the latter form has been popular because of the improved handling properties when the material is chemically sterilized. Caprolactum is partially set by steam sterilization so that bends and kinks made during wrapping are retained, making handling more difficult. Nevertheless, sutures pulled from a germicidal solution through a rubber or plastic cork are not sterile and should not be used, even in the skin. Polymerized caprolactum should not be buried unless steam sterilization is done and unless aseptic conditions are maintained.

Polyester fiber sutures are braided from a synthetic polymer to produce sutures with greater strength that cause less tissue reaction than natural fibers. Multifilament polyester fiber suture has minimal capillarity and withstands sterilization well. In uncoated form, it tends to saw or tear tissues and holds knots poorly. Polyester fiber sutures may be coated with Teflon (Tevdek, Polydek),* silicone (Ticron)† or polybutilate (Ethibond)‡ to reduce drag. The frayed cut ends of sutures cause a local granulomatous response in the tissues. Polyester sutures are suitable for skin and cardiovascular surgery. Large sizes have been implanted as tension sutures during plication of retinacular fascia in dogs. The author has found

this an unsatisfactory use because of the reaction to the frayed ends of the sutures.

Polyethylene and **polypropylene*** are polymerized and extruded as monofilament sutures. They are essentially inert in tissues and retain high tensile strength. Although resembling monofilament nylon in noncapillarity, they are more easily handled and knotted. Nevertheless, multiple throws are recommended for knot security.

Synthetic sutures have wide application in veterinary surgery because of their strength and the relative absence of tissue reaction. All synthetic sutures should be sterile, particularly if buried in the tissues. Buried continuous patterns are suitable for monofilament but not multifilament synthetics. All synthetics knot relatively poorly so that four or more throws or a square knot placed over a surgeon's knot are recommended. In any event, the surgeon should be conscious of the need to place the throws as flat and snug as possible to increase security.

Many sutures are available with swaged-on needles. The limits and testing methods for strength of the needle-suture material attachment have been defined by the U.S. Pharmacopeia (Table 2–4).

CLINICAL USE OF SUTURE MATERIALS

Physical Characteristics

The clinical use of suture materials is dependent on many factors. The physical characteristics of the material are important, as they affect durability, handling, and sterilization characteristics.

Durability should be considered as it relates to the tension of the tissues at the suture line, the healing rate, the strength of the tissue being sutured, and the presence of infection. Monofilament synthetic sutures or stainless steel are preferable to surgical gut in infected or vascular wounds. Synthetic absorbable sutures provide an attractive alternative to many surgeons. It has been suggested that suture strength need not exceed tissue strength, but strength of tissue is poorly defined. Oversized suture

*Deknatel, Inc.
†Davis and Geck
‡Ethicon

*Prolene, Ethicon Co.

TABLE 2–4   U.S.P. Limits for Needle Attachment

USP Sizes Absorbable	Nonabsorbable	Metric Size (Gauge No.)	Limits on Needle Attachment Average* (Kg.)	Individual** (Kg.)
	8–0	0.4	0.050	0.025
	7–0	0.5	0.080	0.040
8–0			0.050†	0.025†
	6–0	0.7	0.17	0.08
7–0			0.080†	0.040†
	5–0	1	0.23	0.11
6–0			0.17†	0.08†
	4–0	1.5	0.45	0.23
5–0			0.23†	0.11†
	3–0	2	0.68	0.34
4–0			0.45†	0.23†
	2–0	3	1.10	0.45
3–0			0.68†	0.34†
	1–0	3.5	1.50	0.45
2–0			1.10†	0.45†
	1	4	1.80	0.60
1–0			1.50†	0.45†
	2 and larger	5 and larger	1.80	0.70
1			1.80†	0.60†
2 and larger		6 and larger	1.8	0.7

*Average of strands.
**If one of five strands breaks prematurely, 10 more must each equal strength.
†Collagen.

material may increase tissue reaction and may knot poorly. Small sutures cause less reaction, form smaller knots, and demand greater attention to detail. Very thin sutures easily cut friable tissue or skin if applied under tension.

The use of suture materials larger than 3–0 in tissues other than fascia of the dog and cat appears unwarranted. Larger sizes are used in fascia (2–0 or 0) and in large animals (0 to 2). The following are general size recommendations for specific tissues: ligation of large vessels and pedicles (0 to 2–0), fascia and dense connective tissue (0 to 3–0 in small animals and 0–2 in large animals), skin and subcutaneous tissue (0 to 4–0), thin skin, skin grafts, and small vessels (3–0 to 4–0), gastrointestinal and urogenital surgery (3–0 to 4–0), vascular sutures (3–0 to 6–0), and nerve sheaths (5–0 to 6–0).

Handling and **knot security** are factors. In many instances, the strongest sutures have the poorest knotting qualities. Each suture is weakest at its tie; none is perfect. No suture is better than the quality, and therefore the technical performance, of the knot.

The importance of *sterilization characteristics* has lessened with the increase in prepackaged, sterilized sutures. Autoclaving is safe, if done no more than three times, on polyester, nylon, polypropylene, and stainless steel. Strength is markedly reduced with multiple autoclaving. Steam sterilization markedly reduces the strengths of nylon, linen, and cotton and is contraindicated for catgut, collagen, fascia lata, polyethylene, and polyglycolic acid.

Gamma irradiation damages polyglycolic acid, polypropylene, linen, and cotton but is acceptable for surgical gut, silk, polyester, nylon, and polyethylene if not repeated more than once. Sterilization with ethylene oxide is safe for all sutures if sufficient aeration time is permitted after sterilization.

Biological Characteristics

The biological characteristics of the suture and the tissues must be considered as a unit because the efficacy of a specific suture material is largely dependent upon the response of tissues.

All sutures produce **tissue reaction** that lasts at least five days. After seven days, the reaction to nonabsorbable sutures becomes minimal. Absorbable sutures behave as nonabsorbable sutures until absorption begins. Monofilament sutures, particularly synthetic ones, produce less tissue reaction than multifilament sutures. A list of sutures in order of increasing intensity of tissue reaction would include synthetic monofilament, synthetic braided, natural braided, and, finally, catgut.

Support of organisms capable of producing *wound infection* is a characteristic of braided and twisted sutures. Introduction of silk, for example, may increase the probability of infection 10,000 times in that 10,000 times the number of organisms that will cause infection in silk suture will be necessary to produce infection when monofilament suture is used. Closer weaves are less likely to support infection but are more difficult to handle.

Chemical composition of the suture also affects the likelihood of infection. Braided nylon is superior to other nonabsorbable multifilament sutures; polyglycolic acid is better than surgical gut in reducing the incidence of wound infection.

The **tissue sutured** is a factor in selection of suture material. Sutures placed near nerves should produce as little inflammation as possible. Small sizes of silk or synthetic sutures should be used. Vascular surgery similarly requires sutures with minimal tissue reaction; silk, coated nylon, and polypropylene are commonly used. Hollow organs have individual characteristics, although they share the possibility of suture extrusion into the lumen. For this reason, chromic surgical gut, polyglycolic acid, and polyglactic acid are recommended for the urinary and biliary tracts. Nonabsorbable sutures may be used in the urinary tract if the lumen is not penetrated by the suture pattern. In gastrointestinal surgery, there is a potential for contamination. Chromic catgut, polypropylene, and monofilament nylon are preferred. Monofilament wire may be used but is difficult to handle. Polyglycolic acid sutures have been used in bowel surgery by some surgeons in spite of their tendency to cut tissues.

Silk may be used to suture the large bowel, but the lumen should be avoided and the surgeon should be aware of the tendency of silk to maintain the growth of organisms.

Monofilament nonabsorbable sutures,

such as stainless steel, nylon, or polypropylene, are used in fascia and tendons in which healing is slow. In skin, noncapillary sutures that produce minimal tissue reaction are less likely to cause scar formation. The size of the scar will also be less if small suture sizes are used. Nevertheless, the size of skin suture is more dependent upon the tension of the closed wound than the propensity for scar formation.

The good surgeon considers both physical and biological characteristics of sutures in establishing his personal preferences. Personal preference is justified because trauma to tissues as a result of poor handling is potentially more detrimental than any available suture.

TYING SUTURES AND LIGATURES

Improvements and refinements in the manufacture and sterilization of surgical materials have provided the surgeon with a wide choice of suture materials. The increased tensile strength and smaller diameter of newer suture materials have reduced the amount of foreign material introduced during the tying of sutures and ligatures. However, the successful use of any of these new materials in tying sutures and ligatures is dependent upon proper knot construction. Each knot must be secure and should hold with proper tension. Speed and dexterity in correct knot tying is an art that is an essential part of the practice of surgery.

The general principles of knot tying apply to all suture materials. The completed knot should be small and the ends cut short to minimize foreign body reaction. The smallest suture material of adequate strength should be used, because knots tied with smaller-sized materials are most secure. In burying knots, suture ends should be cut as short as is practical in order to reduce the amount of suture material left in vivo. Because catgut swells in the tissues, its knot ends should be cut slightly longer. Gentleness is extremely important in tying if one is to prevent suture fracture and tissue damage. Excessive tension must be avoided. If a high degree of tension must be applied to appose tissues or ligate a bleeder, other alternatives should be considered. The knot should be secure so that slippage is impossible but not tied so tightly that tissues strangulate. The exception to this

rule is the application of ligatures for hemostasis; these must be tightly tied around the bleeder. In tying any knot, a sawing or seesaw motion should be avoided, for it weakens the suture materials by wearing or fraying fibers. Clamps or hemostats that will weaken suture material should never be placed on a portion of the suture material that will remain in situ.

After the first loop is made, the suture should not be lifted, nor should uneven pressure be applied to either end, for such pressure will result in loosening of the first throw, thereby producing inadequate tissue apposition or loose ligatures. This loosening can generally be prevented by applying uniform tension and pull to the opposing ends of the suture material rather than by pulling one end more vigorously or rapidly than the other. The square knot will become a half hitch if one end is pulled with greater tension than the other.

Opposing suture ends should be pulled perpendicular to the wound and kept in the same plane. The lifting of one strand or pulling to one side results in half hitches. In instrument ties, the needle holders should remain parallel to the wound and should be moved back and forth perpendicular to it. This also prevents the formation of half hitches.

Since a suture or ligature is virtually useless if the knot slips, the primary objective in tying is to ensure knot security. Of the hundreds of knots available, the square knot is used almost exclusively. Three single reversed throws are generally sufficient to secure knots in suture materials with high coefficients of friction and minimal tension. Synthetic and monofilament suture materials or other sutures with a low coefficient of friction may require four or more throws to prevent knot slippage. In some cases, it may be necessary to overlay a surgeons' knot with a square knot or use two surgeons' knots (double reef knot) to ensure knot security. The surgeons' knot should otherwise be avoided; it is appropriate only when the tissue tension is such that use of the standard square knot would result in poor tissue apposition. The surgeons' knot takes longer to tie and places more suture material in the wound than does the square knot. In addition, it does not permit proper tension upon small vessels because of the bulk of the suture material involved in the first throw. When one is tying knots involving three or more strands of suture material (e.g., at the ends of continuous suture lines), three to four throws are necessary to prevent slippage.

The granny knot, which is made by superimposing one overhand upon another without reversing the second overhand, is not recommended, because it is a slip knot and will loosen. In tying wire sutures, it is especially important to approximate the tissues without constriction or undue tension. A square knot with the cut ends turned over to prevent irritation is recommended. The twisting of wire for knotting is contraindicated in soft tissue, for it results in the strangulation of tissue.

One Hand Square Knot

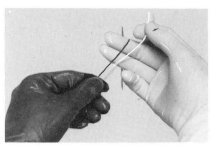

Figure 2–2 The left suture is held in the left hand and passed between the index finger and second finger of the right hand.

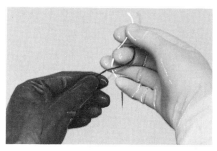

Figure 2–3 The distal phalanx of the second finger of the right hand is flexed to draw the left strand to the right of the right strand. The tip of the second finger is extended so that the white strand is drawn with it through the loop.

Technique for Knots

The step by step illustrations that follow are photographs taken with the camera placed in the position of the surgeon. In each illustration, the left hand is covered with a dark glove and originally holds the dark portion of the suture.

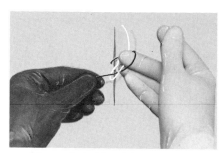

Figure 2–4 The right strand (lighter) is pulled through the loop by the tips of the second and third fingers of the right hand.

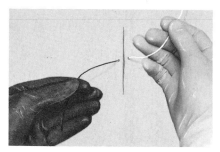

Figure 2–1 The right suture is reflected behind the three fingers of the right (tying) hand and held between the index finger and the thumb.

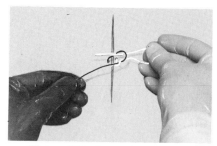

Figure 2–5 The right strand is regrasped with the thumb and fingers.

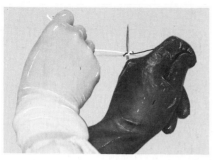

Figure 2–6 The hands are crossed and even tension is applied to the right and left strands.

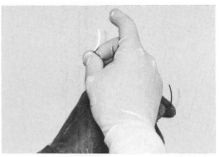

Figure 2–7 The grasp is maintained on the right (white) strand with the thumb and second finger, and the index finger is elevated.

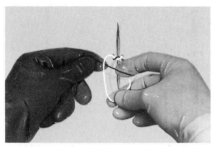

Figure 2–8 The index finger of the right hand is placed between the right and left strands so that the left-hand (dark) strand forms a loop with the right.

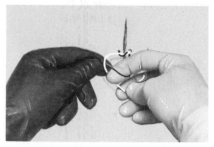

Figure 2–9 The distal phalanx of the right index finger is flexed and then extended to draw the right-hand (white) strand through the loop.

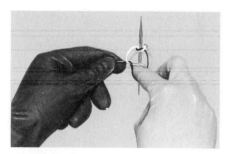

Figure 2–10 The right hand (white) strand is pushed through the loop with the back of the index finger.

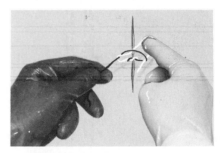

Figure 2–11 The right strand is passed through the loop.

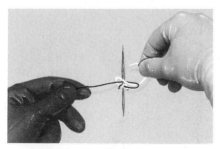

Figure 2–12 The right strand is grasped with the thumb and index finger of the right hand.

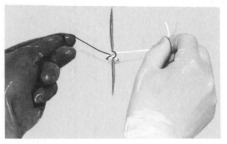

Figure 2–13 Even tension is applied to complete the square knot.

Two Hand Square Knot

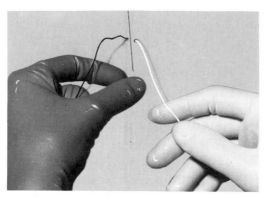

Figure 2–14 The right strand is placed over the extended index finger of the right hand as a bridge; the left strand is held in the palm of the left hand.

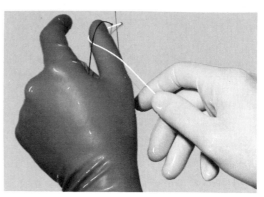

Figure 2–15 The left thumb is passed below and around the right strand; the thumb is then passed to the left of the left strand.

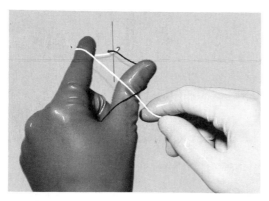

Figure 2–16 The left index finger is introduced with the thumb between the crossed left and right strands.

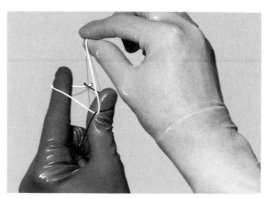

Figure 2–17 The right (white) strand is carried to the left index finger and thumb.

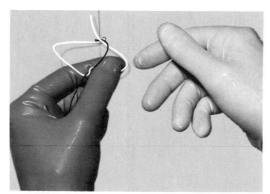

Figure 2–18 The right (white) strand is carried through the loop by the left index finger and thumb and returned to the right hand.

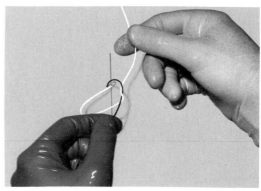

Figure 2–19 The right strand is taken between the right index finger and thumb.

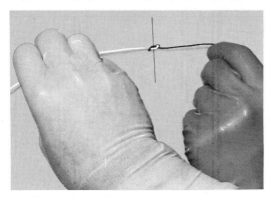

Figure 2–20 The hands are crossed and even tension is applied to the ends.

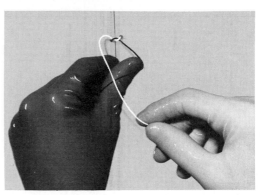

Figure 2–21 The left thumb is placed between the two strands, and a loop is made by the right hand.

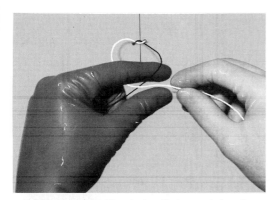

Figure 2–22 The index finger and thumb are joined, and the index finger is passed through the loop to grasp the right (white) strand.

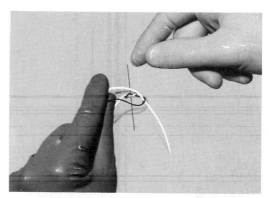

Figure 2–23 The right strand is placed through the loop by the left thumb and index finger.

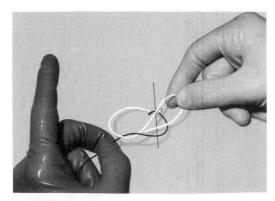

Figure 2–24 The right strand is passed from the left hand to the right thumb and index finger after passing through the loop.

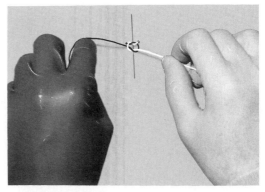

Figure 2–25 Even tension is applied to tighten the square knot.

Instrument Square Knot

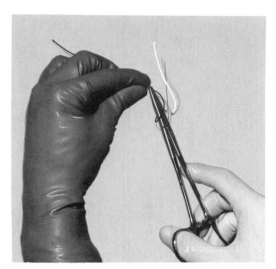

Figure 2–26 The needle holder is placed between the left and right strands, and a loop is formed with the left strand.

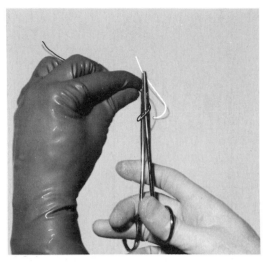

Figure 2–27 The right (short) end is grasped in the needle holder.

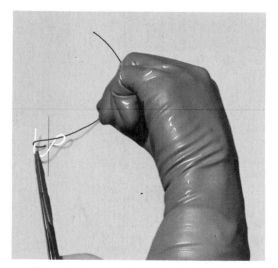

Figure 2–28 The left and right hands are reversed in position, and even tension is applied.

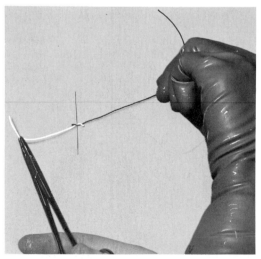

Figure 2–29 The knot is tightened.

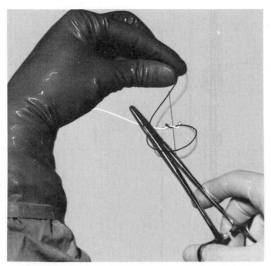

Figure 2–30 A second loop is made by placing the needle holder between the two strands and forming a loop with the long strand.

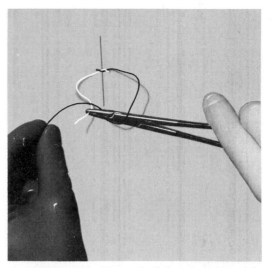

Figure 2–31 The end of the short strand is grasped with the needle holder.

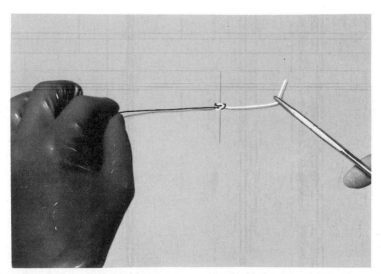

Figure 2–32 The strands are tightened under even tension as they are held close to the incision. The instrument square knot may also be tied by placing the needle holder on the outside of the two strands for each throw. However, placement of the needle holder between the two strands for one throw and exterior to them for the second throw will result in a granny knot.

Instrument Surgeons' Knot

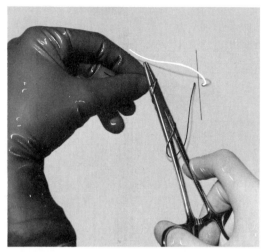

Figure 2–33   The instrument surgeons' knot is tied in much the same fashion as the instrument square knot, but a double loop is placed around the needle holder.

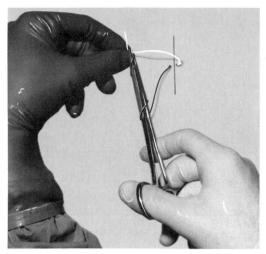

Figure 2–34   The short end is grasped in the needle holder.

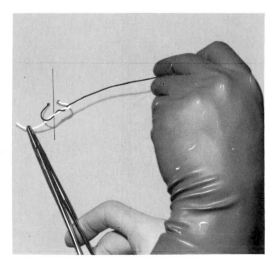

Figure 2–35   The hands are crossed and even tension is applied.

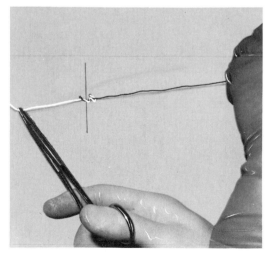

Figure 2–36   The first loop, when tightened, will not slip as readily as it does in the square knot.

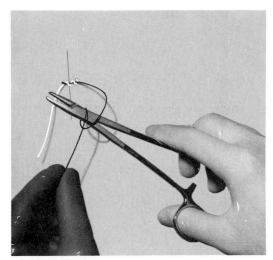

Figure 2–37 The second loop is tied as a single throw around the needle holder, which is placed between the two strands.

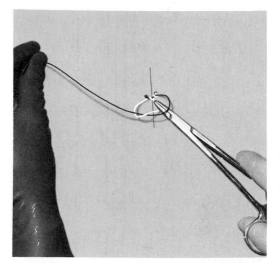

Figure 2–38 The short end is grasped and pulled through the loop.

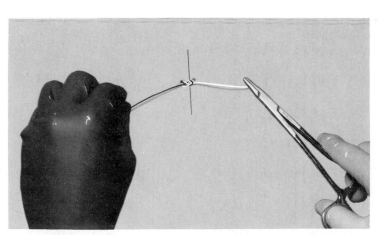

Figure 2–39 Even tension is applied to tighten the knot.

Slip Knots

Slip knots are used for deep ligatures. The use of the slip knot makes possible a tight ligature placed deep from the surface. A square knot may be tied as a slip knot if one end is kept short and an instrument tie is made. A knot may be made to slip by converting the square knot to a half hitch; however, the half hitch will not hold in position as well as a traditional slip knot (Figs. 2–40 to 2–43). The granny has been used because it will slip after the second throw has been made. Extraordinary stresses, likely to produce fraying, are placed upon the suture material when this procedure is used. Mersilene may be made to slip by tying a granny knot. The fixation knot is tied with a true square knot. A square knot may also be used if it is covered with a surgeons' knot. Only the true slip knot is demonstrated.

Traditional Slip Knot

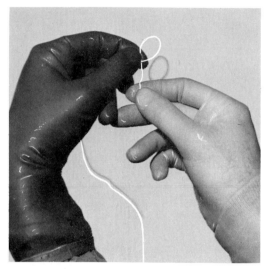

Figure 2–40   A loop is made in the suture.

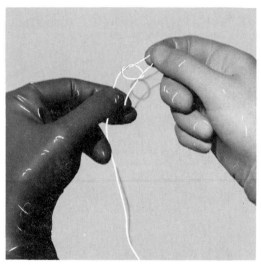

Figure 2–41   The short end is passed through the existing loop to partially complete an overhand throw.

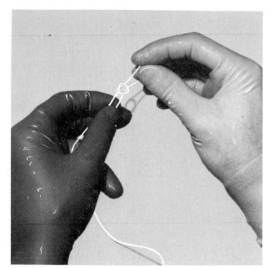

Figure 2–42   The loop is completed and the original tie tightened slightly.

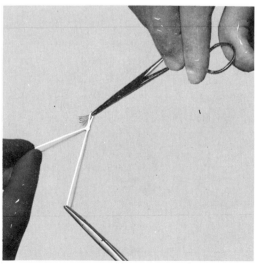

Figure 2–43   The loop is passed over a hemostat to the tissue to be ligated and tightened by traction on the short end with a needle holder.

Double Strand Slip Knot

A firm deep fixation knot may be obtained by passing the center of a suture through the eye of a suture needle. The suture ends are kept short and the looped end is long. The needle is passed through the deepest part of the wound and through the loop of the suture (Fig. 2–44). The suture is pulled tight, and a double-threaded suture pattern is placed continuously from the deep to the superficial layer of the wound. At the superficial end, the knot is tied conventionally.

This technique is particularly useful for repair of diaphragmatic rents in the dog and cat. It provides a secure deep fixation and a double strand of suture.

Miller's Knot

The miller's knot is a simple clove hitch. (Fig. 2–45).

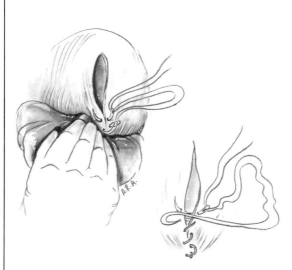

Figure 2–44 Double strand slip knot (diaphragmatic hernia suture).

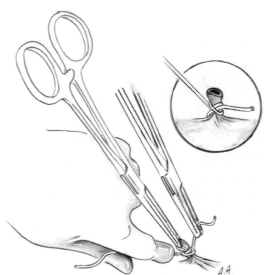

Figure 2–45 Clove hitch or miller's knot.

REFERENCES

Adamsons, R. J., Musco, F., and Enquist, J. F.: Relationship of collagen content to wound strength in normal and scorbutic animals. Surg. Gynecol. Obstet., 1964, *119*:323.

Adler, R. H., Montes, M., Doyer, R., and Harrod, D.: A comparison of reconstituted collagen suture and catgut suture for colon anastomoses. Surg. Gynecol. Obstet., 1967, *124*:1245.

Alexander, J. W., Kaplan, J. Z., and Altemeier, W. A.: Role of suture materials in the development of wound infection. Ann. Surg., 1967, *192*:165.

Baker, R., Maxted, W. C., and DiPasquale, N.: Regeneration of transitional epithelium of the human bladder after total surgical excision for recurrent multiple bladder cancer. J. Urol., 1965, *93*:593.

Bartone, F. F. and Shires, T. K.: The reaction of kidney and bladder tissue to catgut and reconstituted collagen sutures. Surg. Gynecol. Obstet., 1969, *128*:1221.

Bartone, F. F. and Shires, T. K.: The reaction of the urinary tract to catgut and reconstituted collagen sutures. J. Urol., 1969, *101*:411.

Bergenholtz, A. and Isaksson, B.: Tissue reaction in the oral mucosa to cutgut, silk, and mersilene sutures. Odontol. Revy., 1967, *18*:237.

Bohne, A. W., Osborn, R. W., and Hettle, P. J.: Regeneration of the urinary bladder in the dog, following total cystectomy. Surg. Gynecol. Obstet., 1955, *100*:259.

Botsford, T. W.: The tensile strength of sutured skin wounds during healing. Surg. Gynecol. Obstet., 1941, *72*:690.

Cocke, W. M.: Dexon — a new suture material: Its use in plastic surgery. South. Med. J., 1972, *65*:629.

Cushing, H. and Bovie, W. T.: Electrosurgery as an aid to the removal of intracranial tumors. Surg. Gynec. Obstet., 1928, *47*:751.

Davis and Geck, Inc.: *Suture Manual.* Pearl River, N.Y.: American Cyanamid Co., 1971.

Echeverria, A. and Jimeniz, J.: Evaluation of an absorbable synthetic suture material. Surg. Gynecol. Obstet., 1970, *131*:1.

Ethicon, Inc.: *Manual of Surgical Procedures and Surgical Knots.* Somerville, N.J.: Ethicon, Inc., 1961.

Everett, W. G.: Suture materials in general surgery. Prog. Surg., 1970, 8:14.

Forrester, J. C.: Suture materials. Nursing Mirror, 1975, *140*:48.

Gaskin, E. R. and Childers, M. D., Jr.: Increased granuloma formation from absorbable sutures. J.A.M.A., 1913, *185*:212.

Gibson, T. and Kenedi, R. M.: Factors affecting the mechanical characteristics of human skin. In *Repair and Regeneration*, ed. Dunphy, J. E. and Van Winkle, W., Jr. New York: McGraw-Hill Book Co., 1969.

Gray, F. J. and Herbert, C.: An experimental study of the influence of selected suture materials on healing of aponeurotic tissue. Aust. J. Surg., 1967, *137*:41.

Greene, J. A., and Knecht, C. D.: Healing of sharp and electroincisions in dogs. A comparative study. J. Vet. Surg., 9(2):42–48, 1980.

Grier, R. L.: Surgical Sutures — Part 1: A Review. Iowa State University Veterinarian, 3, 1971.

Grier, R. L.: Surgical Sutures — Part 2: Indications for Different Suture Material and Comparable Cost. Iowa State University Veterinarian 2, 1972.

Halsted, W. S.: Ligature and suture material. J.A.M.A., 1913, *60*:1119.

Herrmann, J. B., Kelly, R. J., and Higgins, G. A.: Polyglycolic acid sutures. Arch. Surg., 1970, *100*:486.

Herrmann, J. B.: Changes in tensile strength and knot security of surgical sutures in vivo. Arch. Surg., 1973, *106*:707–710.

Homsy, C. A., McDonald, K. E., and Akers, W. W.: Surgical suture — canine tissue interaction for six common suture types. J. Biomed. Mat. Res., 1968, 2:215.

Howes, E. L.: Effects of suture material on the tensile strength of wound repair. Ann. Surg., 1933, 98:153.

Howes, E. L.: The immediate strength of the sutured wound. Surg., 1940, 7:24.

Jenkins, H. P. and Hrdina, L. S.: Absorption of surgical gut (catgut). I. Decline in tensile strength in the tissues. Arch. Surg., 1937, *34*:209.

Katz, A. R. and Turner,, R. J.: Evaluation of tensile and absorption properties of polyglycolic acid sutures. Surg., Gynecol. Obstet., 1970, *131*:701.

Kreshon, M. J., Lymberis, M. N., and Leonard, R.: Collagen sutures in cataract surgery: An evaluation of 400 cases. Trans. Am. Acad. Ophthalmol. Otolaryngol. 1966, *70*:959.

Lichtenstein, I. L., Herzikoff, S., Shore, J. M., Jiron, M. W., Stuart, S., and Mizuno, L.: The dynamics of wound healing. Surg., Gynecol. Obstet., 1970, *130*:685.

Lilly, G. E., Cutcher, J. L., Jones, J. C., and Armstrong, J. H.: Reaction of oral tissues to suture materials — IV. Oral Surg., 1972, *33*:152.

Ludewig, R. M., Rudolph, L. E., and Wangensteen, S. L.: Reduction of experimental wound infection with iodized gut sutures. Surg., Gynecol. Obstet. 1971, *133*:946.

Madsen, E. T.: An experimental and clinical evaluation of surgical suture materials. Surg., Gynecol. Obstet. 1953, 97:73.

Mead, W. H. and Ochsner, A.: The relative value of catgut, silk, linen, and cotton as suture materials. Surg., 1940, 7:485.

Mendoza, C. B., Jr., Watne, A. L., Grace, J. E., and Moore, G. E.: Wire versus silk: Choice of surgical wound closure in patients with cancer. Am. J. Surg., 1966, *112*:839.

Owens, G. and Rubbra, J.: The effect of various suture materials in wound healing. J. Kans. Med. Soc., 1946, *47*:300.

Partipilo, A. V.: *Surgical Technique and Principles of Operative Surgery*, 6th Ed. Philadelphia: Lea and Febiger, 1957.

Postlethwait, R. W.: Long-term comparative study of nonabsorbable sutures. Ann. Surg., 1970, *171*:892.

Postlethwait, R. W.: Tissue reaction to surgical suture. In *Repair and Regeneration*, ed. Dunphy, J. E. and VanWinkle, H. W., Jr. New York: McGraw-Hill Book Co., Inc., 1969.

Postlethwait, R. W., Schauble, J. F., Dillon, M. L., and Freeman, J.: Wound healing. I. Comparison of heat and irradiation sterilized surgical sutures. Arch Surg., 1959, 78:958.

Postlethwait, R. W., Schauble, J. E., Dillon, M. L., and Morgan, J.: Evaluation of surgical suture material. Surg., Gynecol. Obstet., 1959, *108*:555.

Postlethwait, R. W., et al.: Polyglycolic acid sutures. Arch. Surg., 1970, *100*:486–490.

Preston, D. J.: The effects of sutures on the strength of healing wounds. Am. J. Surg., 1940, *49*:56.

Rhoads, J. E., Hotenstein, H. F., and Hudson, I. F.: The decline in strength of catgut after exposure to living tissues. Arch. Surg., 1937, *34*:209.

Sandberg, N.: On the healing of wounds in rats during the period of cicatrization. Acta. Chir. Scand., 1963, *126*:294.

Salthouse, T. N., Williams, J. A., and Willigan, D. A.: Relationship of cellular enzyme activity to catgut and collagen suture absorption. Surg. Gynecol. Obstet., 1969, *129*:691.

Schechter, D. C.: The history of the evolution of methods of hemostasis and the study of blood coagulation. In *Surgical Bleeding – Handbook for Medicine, Surgery and Specialities.* Ulen, A. W. and Gollub, S. S. eds. New York: McGraw-Hill Book Co., 1966.

Scheinin, T. M. and Viljanto, J.: Bursting pressure of healing gastrointestinal wounds in the rat. Ann. Med. Exp. Fenn, 1966, *44*:49.

Scholz, K. C., Lewis, R. C., and Bateman, R. O.: Clinical failure of polyglycolic acid surgical suture. Surg., Gynecol. Obstet., 1952, *135*:525.

Silvennoineu, E.: Concretements resulting from suture materials in the biliary tract. Ann. Chir. Gyne., Fenn. (Suppl), 1970, *59*:169.

Stashak, T. S. and Yturraspe, D. J.: Consideration for selection of suture materials. J. Vet. Surg., 1978, 7:48.

Thoenes, L. A.: The properties of catgut sutures sterilized by heat, ethylene oxide, and electron beams, J. Int. Coll. Surg., 1964, *42*:382.

Troup, S. B. and Schwartz, S. I.: Thermal agents. In *Principles of Surgery.* ed. Schwartz, S. I. New York: McGraw-Hill Book Co., 1969. pp. 106–107.

Udupa, K. N. and Chansouria, J. P. N.: Studies on

wound healing. II. Role of suture materials in the healing of skin wounds. Ind. J. Med. Res., 1969, 57:442.

United States Pharmacopeia, 19th Revision, U.S. Pharmacopeial Convention, Inc., Rockville, Md., 1975, pp. 484, 665.

Usher, F. C., Allen, J. E., Crosthwait, R. W., and Cogan, J. E.: Polypropylene monofilament, a new biologically inert suture for closing contaminated wounds. J.A.M.A., 1962, 179:780.

VanWinkle, W., Jr. and Hastings, J. C.: Considerations in the choice of suture material for various tissues. Surg., Gynecol. Obstet., 1972, 135:113.

VanWinkle, W.: The tensile strength of wounds and factors that influence it. Surg., Gynecol. Obstet. 1969, 129:819.

Walter, C. W.: *The Aseptic Treatment of Wounds.* New York: The Macmillan Co., 1948.

Walter, C. W., and Arlein, M. S.: Aseptic technique in veterinary surgery. J.A.V.M.A., 1943, 102:41.

Welser, J. R.: Suture materials. In *Fundamental Techniques in Veterinary Surgery.* ed. Knecht, C. D., et al. Philadelphia: W. B. Saunders Co., 1975, pp. 20–25.

Yudofsky, S. C., and Scott, F. B.: Urolithiasis on suture materials: Its importance, pathogenesis, and prophylaxis; an introduction to the monofilament Teflon suture. J. Urol., 1969, 102:745.

3

SUTURE PATTERNS

3

SUTURE PATTERNS

INTRODUCTION

A number of surgical suture patterns are used in man and animals. For purposes of categorization, the suture patterns are described as *continuous* or *interrupted.* Continuous sutures are not cut short or quickly severed; they run from the point of origin to some relatively distant end point. They incorporate numerous bites in the tissue. Interrupted sutures are tied and cut after one or two passages through the tissue. Lembert and Cushing sutures are examples of the continuous suture; horizontal and vertical mattress sutures are two types of interrupted sutures. There are simple continuous and simple interrupted sutures as well. Suture patterns need not be described exclusively as continuous or interrupted. Indeed, they may be divided into the *simple* and *mattress* categories. The simple type of suture is one that directly apposes adjacent tissues by a single passage through the tissue on each side of the incision. Mattress sutures are designed to withstand added tensions. Mattress sutures incorporate a small mass of tissue on each side of the incision.

Suture patterns may additionally be classified as everting, inverting, and apposing. The latter suture is designed to bring the tissues in direct apposition. Everting sutures tend to turn the tissue edges outward (away from the patient and toward the surgeon). Inverting sutures turn the tissue inward toward the patient or toward the lumen of a viscus. The advantages and uses of the various suture patterns will be discussed individually.

INTERRUPTED SUTURES

Simple Interrupted

The primary advantage of the interrupted suture is its ability to maintain strength and tissue position should part of the suture line fail. Each suture in the interrupted pattern is individually tied and severed distal to the knot; each suture is therefore a unit and not entirely subject to the strength of the adjacent sutures. The technique for the individual sutures is easy and rapid. The disadvantages of interrupted sutures are the greater amount of suture material used, the overall time involved in tying and cutting additional knots, and the presence of additional amounts of suture material in the tissues in the form of knots. Frequently, these knots may be palpable for some time after surgery. In addition, the pattern has minimal holding power against stress.

The simple interrupted suture is made by directing the needle through the tissue approximately 2 to 3 mm (⅛") lateral to the incision line. The suture is inserted through the tissue on one side, passed through that on the opposite side, taking the same amount of tissue in a single bite, and tied. The knot should be offset, so as not to rest upon the incision, and the ends should be cut. The next simple interrupted suture is placed approximately 0.5 cm from the first (Fig. 3–1). The surgeon should take advan-

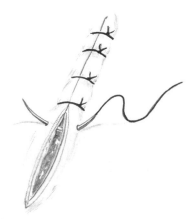

Figure 3–1 Simple interrupted suture pattern.

tage of the field of incision and his own dexterity by placing sutures from right to left in a horizontal incision if he is right-handed, and from left to right if he is left-handed. Whatever hand they favor, all surgeons should suture a vertical incision from the end most distal toward the end most proximal. The simple interrupted suture is an apposing suture if properly applied, but excessive tension will generally cause inversion. Inversion of the skin should never be allowed; eversion would be preferable. Inverting simple interrupted skin sutures should be converted to everting sutures before a bandage is applied.

Horizontal Mattress Suture

The horizontal mattress suture is a tension suture. It is used where relative speed is desired but the need for a larger tissue mass within the suture is apparent. It is particularly useful in suturing the skin of the dog; the horse; and the cow. In making the horizontal mattress suture, the surgeon introduces the needle 2 to 3 mm to the right of the incision (if he is right-handed). The needle is passed angularly through the tissue below the edge of the tissue plane, crosses the incision line, and exits in an angular pattern on the opposite side. The suture is advanced approximately 8 mm and is introduced from the left side, crossing the incision line to the right side. The suture is tied on the right side (Fig. 3–2). The advantages of the horizontal mattress suture are twofold: It involves a small amount of suture material and it can be rapidly applied. In addition, a tension type of suture is

obtained. The primary disadvantage of the horizontal mattress suture is the relative difficulty of applying it in skin without causing excessive eversion. The fact that the pattern is so difficult for the novice to apply properly makes it an excellent teaching tool requiring total concentration on technique. If the mattress suture is applied so that it angles through the skin and passes just below the dermis — and if the incision is just tight enough for the skin edges to meet — eversion is less likely to occur (Fig. 3–3). Depending on the subject and the

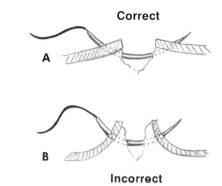

Correct

A

B

Incorrect

Figure 3–3 Positioning of the horizontal mattress suture.

tissues to be sutured, the horizontal mattress sutures are usually separated by a 4 mm space.

Vertical Mattress Suture

The vertical mattress suture is also a tension suture. It is stronger in tissues under tension than is the horizontal mattress suture. The disadvantages of the vertical mattress suture are that it requires an increased amount of suture material and is time-consuming to apply. The vertical mattress suture is introduced approximately 8 mm from the incision on one side, passed across the incision line, and made to exit at an equal distance on the opposite side of the incision. The needle is then reversed and returned to the original side by passing 4 mm or less from the incision on each side. The knot is tied on the side of origin (Fig. 3–4). The sutures should be placed approximately 5 mm apart. There is little eversion, because the returning suture is placed close to the incision line.

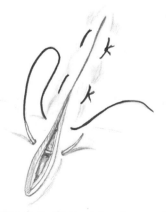

Figure 3–2 Horizontal mattress pattern.

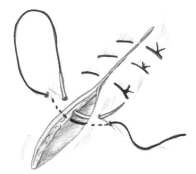

Figure 3–4   Vertical mattress suture.

The Cross Mattress Suture (The X-Mattress Suture)

A modification of the mattress suture is the cross mattress suture (the X-mattress suture). This suture is applied as if it were two simple interrupted sutures joined together. The needle is introduced on one side 3 to 4 mm from the incision and is passed to a corresponding point on the opposite side. The needle is then advanced approximately 5 mm and is passed across the incision line without entering the tissues. A second passage is made through the tissues parallel to the first passage. The suture origin on one side is tied to the contralateral end on the tissue surface. A figure X is obtained (Fig. 3–5). The cross

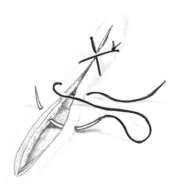

Figure 3–5   Cross mattress suture (or X-mattress suture).

mattress is a tension suture that has the advantage of bringing tissues into apposition, which is particularly useful in suturing stumps. Amputations of the tail and digits of dogs tend to result in flaps of skin that open rather than join. The vertical mattress pattern may be used to close such stumps

effectively but requires twice as many sutures as the cross mattress pattern. Cross mattress sutures provide strength and prevent eversion.

Crushing or Gambee Suture

Crushing sutures are useful in intestinal anastomoses, in which a single-layer interrupted closure is desired. Experimental studies in the dog and cat indicate that crushing sutures produce minimal leakage and good apposition of viscera with large lumen size. The suture is introduced much like a simple interrupted suture, passing from serosa through muscularis and mucosa to the lumen. The suture is returned from the lumen through the mucosa to the muscularis before it crosses the incision or the site of anastomosis. The needle is introduced in the muscularis on the opposite side and is continued through the mucosa to the lumen. It is then reintroduced through mucosa, muscularis, and serosa to exit at the external surface. The beginning and end are tied tightly so that the suture impresses itself on the bowel tissue (Fig. 3–6). The

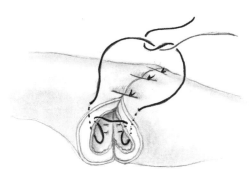

Figure 3–6   Crushing or gambee suture.

pattern tends to reduce the passage of fluid from the lumen to the serosa along the suture, which occurs in most through-and-through sutures (this characteristic is known as the wick tendency). In the dog and the cat, the crushing suture has caused minimal stenosis, adhesions, and infection.

Burying the Knot

In certain suture patterns, the knot should be buried beneath the tissue surface to prevent excessive irritation. Catgut sutures of subcutaneous and subcuticular tissues should be buried; it they are not, the presence of a large knot below the skin may cause excessive pressure and local necrosis of the skin. The knot may be buried by introducing the needle deep in the subcutaneous tissues and passing the suture toward the dermis. The exit point of the suture is the incision line ventral to the dermis (Fig. 3–7). The suture is then passed across the

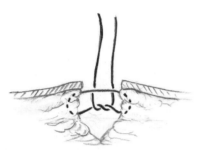

Figure 3–7 Burying the knot.

incision line, introduced in the subcutaneous tissue close to the dermis, incorporating subcutaneous tissues, and is recovered deep in the incision line. The beginning and end are knotted deep in the tissues.

CONTINUOUS SUTURES

Continuous sutures are those that are neither knotted nor cut after each introduction or pair of introductions through the tissue. The advantages of the continuous suture line are ease of application, minimal use of suture material, minimal amount of knots, and ease of removal. In addition, there is more complete tissue apposition. Where simple interrupted sutures may cause a curtaining effect between sutures, a continuous pattern will firmly appose the adjacent tissues and will prevent fluid or tissue leakage through the incision line. The primary disadvantage of the continuous suture pattern is the dependence of the whole pattern on each of its parts. Slippage of either the beginning or end knot is likely to cause failure of the entire suture line. Particular attention must be paid to the integrity of the suture material and the knots when continuous sutures are used. The surgeon suturing in a continuous line

should grasp catgut sutures with forceps *only* when tying a knot. Any other compression with forceps causes a loss of strength, which may result in the loss of the suture pattern.

Simple Continuous Suture

The simple continuous suture consists of a series of simple interrupted sutures that are tied at the beginning and end but are continuous between these two points. A simple interrupted suture is placed and knotted, but only the short, or non-needle, end is cut. The end with the needle is advanced and introduced through the tissue perpendicular to the incision line. No tying is done as the suture is again advanced and reintroduced in the same direction as the previous sutures. The suture pattern that results has a suture perpendicular to the incision line below the tissue and advancing forward above it (Fig. 3–8). At the end of

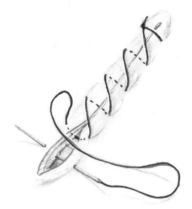

Figure 3–8 Simple continuous suture.

the incision line, or a distance usually not exceeding 13 cm (5″), the suture is tied with three single throws. When a swaged-on needle is used, the needle end of the suture is tied to the last available loop of suture material that is exterior to the tissues (Fig 3–9). The procedure differs if a needle with an eye is used; the needle is advanced through the tissues, and the short end of the suture is held on the proximal end of the needle passage. A loop of suture is pulled through with the needle, and this loop is tied to the single end on the contralateral side (Fig. 3–10). The knot is tied, and the suture material is cut close on the knot. A

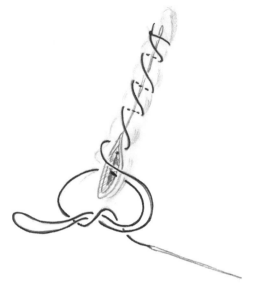

Figure 3–9 Ending a continuous suture with a swaged-on needle.

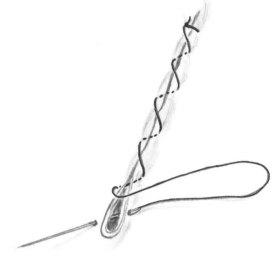

Figure 3–11 Running suture.

modification of the simple continuous suture is the *running suture*. The running suture is a simple continuous suture in which both the deep and superficial portions advance rather than the deep portion passing perpendicular to the incision line (Fig. 3–11). The result is a basting stitch. The running stitch allows the surgeon to advance the suture somewhat faster than does the simple continuous suture; nevertheless, regularity in stitching (i.e., a symmetrical pattern) is more difficult to achieve.

Simple continuous sutures are generally used in tissues that require minimal holding but maximal tissue apposition. The peritoneum in the dog is adequately closed with the simple continuous suture; the suture tends to create an air- and liquid-tight seal that prevents passage of even minimal quantities of omentum through the incision line.

The simple continuous suture is also quite useful in the closure of subcutaneous tissues and fascia in non-tension planes. The knot may be buried with simple continuous and running sutures. The first pass is begun deep in the tissues and is directed toward the surface. The needle is reinserted from the surface and is directed to the deep tissues on the opposite side. The end of the suture should be held toward the open portion of the incision line rather than toward the starting point of the sutures. The needle is passed toward the short end, and a knot is tied deep in the tissues (Fig. 3–12). The same pattern is applied at the opposite end of the incision. Before the last suture is placed, the needle is inserted from superficial to deep in the tissues, and a loop of suture is lifted from the incision line. The needle is then introduced from deep in the tissues to superficial on one side, allowed to cross the incision, and inserted from superficial to deep in the tissue toward the loop (Fig. 3–13). The end of the suture is then tied to the deep loop.

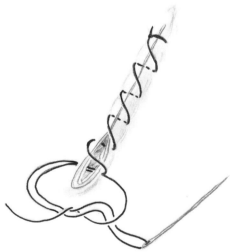

Figure 3–10 Ending a continuous suture with an eyed needle.

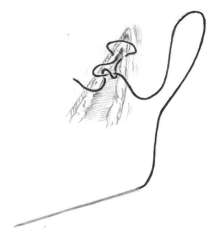

Figure 3-12 Buried knot (beginning).

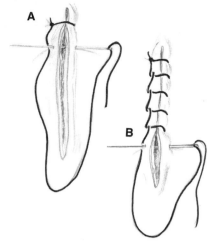

Figure 3–14 Ford interlocking suture.

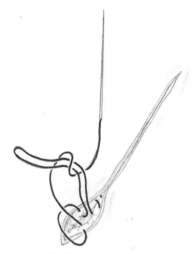

Figure 3–13 Buried knot (ending).

Ford Interlocking Suture

The Ford interlocking suture is a modification of the simple continuous suture. The pattern is continuous, but each passage through the tissue is partially locked. The needle is inserted on one side of the incision and is passed as a simple interrupted suture to the opposite side. The origin is then tied, and the short end of the suture is cut. The needle is advanced, a loop is formed, and the needle is passed perpendicularly through the tissues in the same direction. After the needle is passed from the tissues, it is drawn through the preformed loop and tightened (Fig. 3–14). The pattern through the tissues and loop is repeated, locking each stitch, until the end of the

pattern is reached. In terminating a lock stitch, the needle should be introduced in the opposite direction from that previously used, and the end should be held on the side of insertion (Fig. 3–15). A loop of suture, formed on the side opposite that of introduction, is tied to the single end (Fig. 3–16). The advantage of the lock stitch is its greater stability in the event of partial failure: failure of a knot or of a portion of the suture line does not necessarily result in failure of the entire line. In addition, a greater degree of tissue stability results, because tissues incorporated in adjacent lock stitches are not likely to slide. The disadvantage of the Ford interlocking suture is that a large amount of suture material will be used and left in the incision area. If it is applied to skin, the suture is slightly difficult to remove.

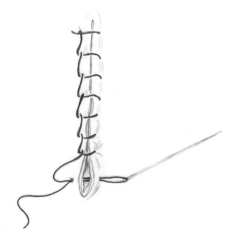

Figure 3–15 Final stitch in Ford interlocking suture.

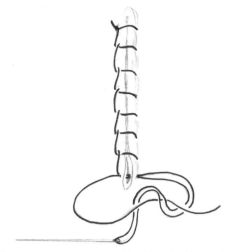

Figure 3–16 Final tie in Ford interlocking suture.

Lembert Suture

The Lembert suture is an inverting continuous vertical mattress suture. It is used primarily to close hollow viscera that require inversion and a firm mattress pattern.

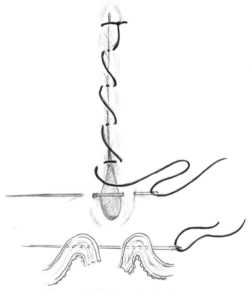

Figure 3–17 Lembert suture.

The suture is applied from outside the lumen, with the needle passing through the serosa and muscularis and returning through muscularis and serosa to the area outside the viscera on the same side of the incision. The needle is then passed across the incision to the opposite side and is introduced on the serosal surface adjacent to the incision. It is passed through serosa and muscularis and is continued to the distant serosa. The beginning and end are tied. The short end of the suture is cut, and the needle is advanced (Fig. 3–17) so that this vertical mattress pattern may be repeated around the viscera and tied.

A Lembert suture with only two parallel but reversing passages through the tissue (interrupted inverting mattress pattern) is called a *Halsted* suture (Fig. 3–18).

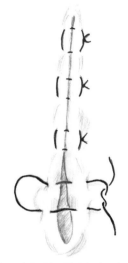

Figure 3–18 Halsted suture.

Connell and Cushing Sutures

The Connell suture enters the lumen, but the Cushing suture passes only to the submucosa. Each is an inverting continuous horizontal mattress pattern. The Connell suture is generally begun with a single inverting vertical mattress suture. From its point of exit the needle is then advanced parallel to the incision and is introduced into the serosa, passing through the muscular and mucosal surfaces and extending into the lumen. From the lumen the needle is advanced further along the incision (still parallel to it) and is returned through mucosa, muscularis, and serosa to the same side of the incision (Fig. 3–19). Once outside the viscera, the needle and suture are passed across the incision and are introduced at a point that corresponds (in distance from the incision) to the exit point on the contralateral side. This stitch is introduced so that the

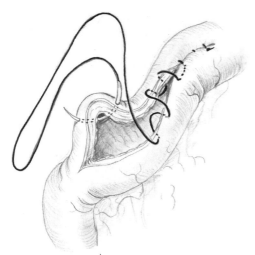

Figure 3–19 Connell suture.

each suture pattern inverts the tissue, but more tissue is inverted in the Lembert pattern.) The Connell pattern generally should be applied with a covering suture, in order to prevent penetration of a single suture from the serosa to the lumen.

Modifications of Lembert and Cushing patterns are used to close the stump of hollow viscera. The *Parker-Kerr* suture consists of a single layer of Cushing pattern covered by a layer of Lembert (Figs. 3–21 to 3–23). This double inversion is used for infected uterine stumps and certain bowel closures. The obvious disadvantage of the

suture can cross the incision perpendicularly. The needle is reinserted through serosa, muscularis, and mucosa, advanced within the lumen parallel to the incision, and exited again. When tightened, the visible portions of the suture are perpendicular to the incision line. The suture is not tied until the incision is completely stitched.

The Cushing differs from the Connell in that the suture does not pass into the lumen but extends only to the submucosal area. The direction of pattern in the two sutures is the same (Fig. 3–20). (In addition,

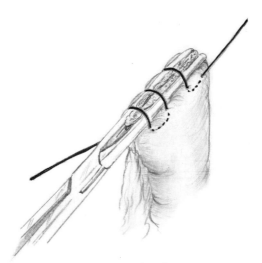

Figure 3–21 First layer in a Parker-Kerr suture.

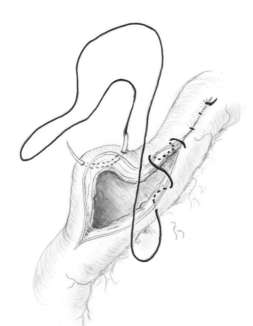

Figure 3–20 Cushing suture.

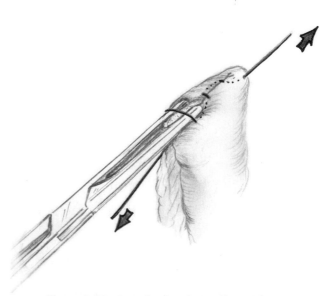

Figure 3–22 Inversion in a Parker-Kerr suture.

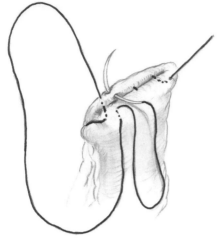

Figure 3–23 Second layer in a Parker-Kerr suture.

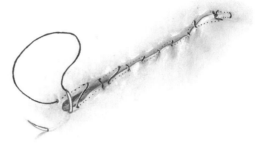

Figure 3-24 Guard suture.

Parker-Kerr closure is the presence of an outer layer that communicates between the serosa and the lumen. For practical purposes, the suture pattern should be reversed, with the Lembert pattern applied first and the Cushing suture applied afterward. The Parker-Kerr pattern is useful if the first layer is applied over Rochester-Carmalt forceps and is not tied. The Carmalt forceps are then gently withdrawn as the suture is pulled in both directions. This permits inversion of the stump without opening the lumen, thereby preventing contamination and any loss of contents. A second layer of Cushing suture is then applied.

Another modification of suture patterns is to apply a Cushing over a Connell pattern. Alternatively, one may apply two Cushing lines.

Modified Cushing Pattern (Guard Pattern)

The Guard pattern is a modification of the Cushing pattern. It is continuous and inverting. It is used in closing incisions in the rumen, intestine, and uterus. The needle does not penetrate the lumen of the viscera.

The pattern is begun at a point slightly above the end of the incision (Fig. 3–24). In large animals, the needle is inserted 12 to 20 mm from the incision and is carried through the tissue parallel to the line of incision. It exits above the initial penetration and is moved across the extended line of incision and is reinserted for a contralateral parallel bite. It is tied across the incision, and the needle is reinserted slightly above and lateral to the knot. After the needle is directed distally parallel to the incision, the suture is continued as a Cushing pattern. At the end of the incision, the needle is passed downward, leaving a trailing end. The needle then crosses above the incision and is inserted retrograde on the other side. It is tied across the incision to the trailing end.

This pattern causes inversion and better sealing of the incision ends than does the standard Cushing suture. A large roll at the bottom of the incision, which would allow escape of fluids, is avoided.

Continuous Everting Mattress Suture

The continuous everting mattress suture is used for skin closure when a continuous suture is acceptable, a degree of eversion is not objectionable, and increased tension is desired. The pattern is developed as interrupted horizontal mattress sutures are applied continuously. The suture pattern is begun with a simple interrupted suture; this suture is then tied and the short end is cut. The suture is advanced approximately 5 mm, and a second pass is made through the tissue perpendicular to the incision. Upon exiting from the tissue, the needle is advanced 7 to 8 mm and is reinserted perpendicular to the incision line in the contralateral direction. The resultant suture pattern is continuous and passes through the tissue perpendicular to the incision but parallel to the tissue on alternate sides external to the incision (Fig. 3–25). The continuous everting mattress suture is used for skin closures in which rapid closure is desired.

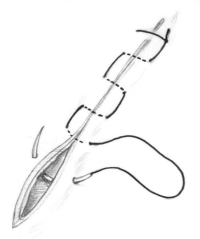

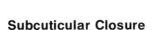

Figure 3–25 Continuous everting mattress suture.

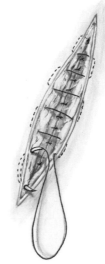

Figure 3–26 Subcuticular closure.

Subcuticular Closure

Subcuticular closure may be used in place of skin sutures to eliminate scars that form around sutures in the skin. The suture pattern is continuous — and has all of the faults of continuous sutures. It *is* rapid and utilizes very little suture material, but it does not have the strength of normal skin sutures; in domestic animals, it is subject to removal by biting, licking, or scratching. The suture is begun by burying the knot, with the beginning bite being taken in the dermis. The suture is passed beneath the dermis on the original side to the dermis on the opposite side, and the knot is tied deep in the tissues. The inverted continuous vertical mattress pattern is continued to the other end of the incision, and a knot is buried at the opposite end. Catgut or other absorbable material must be used when the suture is to be buried. A subcuticular closure may also be made in a horizontal mattress pattern with the needle crossing perpendicular to the incision but advancing in the underside of the dermis parallel to the incision (Fig. 3–26).

Subcuticular suture patterns can be stitched with nonabsorbable suture materials. Of course, an additional step is necessary to ensure the removal of the suture material. To start the pattern, a small simple interrupted suture is begun at one end of the incision, and the short end of the suture material is cut. The suture is inserted through the skin and is applied in a continuous horizontal mattress pattern in the underside of the dermis from the beginning of the incision to its opposite end. The passages of suture between bites in the dermis should be truly perpendicular. At the end, the subcuticular suture is again inserted through the skin, and another perpendicular passage is made in the skin from the outside surface (epidermis). The suture is tied and the ends are cut. When the skin is healed, the one end of the suture is pulled and cut on the knot. The other end may then be loosened from the skin and gently pulled intact from the subcuticular area. The procedure for application is simple, but that for removal may be difficult and painful. The subcuticular suture pattern with nonabsorbable suture appears adequate for short incisions (2.5 to 5 cm).

Subcutaneous Closure

Subcutaneous tissues may be apposed with simple interrupted, simple continuous, or horizontal mattress suture patterns. The first type is more secure but takes more time and places more knots in the subcutaneous tissues. Each suture should be placed with the knot buried. A horizontal mattress pattern, as previously described for subcuticular closure (Fig. 3–26), may be placed without insertion of the suture into the dermis. The disadvantage is that a pocket is likely to result in the tissues deep to the suture pattern.

A simple continuous subcutaneous pattern is preferred because it is fast, easy to

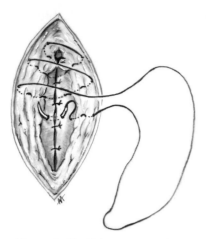

Figure 3–27 Subcutaneous closure.

sponge on the incision. Excessive pressure may cause necrosis.

Quilled sutures are vertical mattress sutures with everting characteristics. They incorporate a rubber, plastic, or gauze tube in the external loop on each side of the incision (Fig. 3–28). The suture is begun

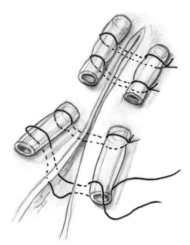

Figure 3–28 Quilled suture.

apply, and obliterates dead space. The suture is begun by burying the knot (Fig. 3–12). The needle is inserted from the deep layers of subcutaneous tissue toward the skin but does not penetrate the dermis and returns to a similar deep contralateral location. After knotting, the suture is placed from a deep to superficial direction, and the needle is regrasped. The pattern is continued by a series of loops that incorporate several subcutaneous tissue bites on one side, a deep fascial bite, and several subcutaneous bites on the opposite side (Fig. 3–27). Incorporation of large amounts of tissue is counterproductive, causing eversion and separation of the skin, and is unnecessary for apposition of tissues. The loops are placed 0.7 to 1.5 cm apart, and the suture line is terminated by burying the knot (Fig. 3–13).

Absorbable sutures are commonly used for subcutaneous closure. The pattern should be tied, cut, and restarted in incisions longer than 12 cm.

SPECIAL TENSION SUTURE PATTERNS

Stent and Quilled Sutures

The Stent and quilled suture patterns are designed for wounds that subject normal sutures to excessive pressure and tension. Each is applied to the skin in areas of extreme stress in addition to appositional sutures. A Stent suture is made by incorporating sterile gauze sponge in a large, simple interrupted suture that presses the

distant from the incision and is passed through the skin and subcutaneous tissues, crossing the incision line. It exits far from the incision and on the opposite side. It is looped while it is external to the skin and is reinserted at a point that is closer to the incision than is the point of exit. The suture then passes through the skin and subcutaneous tissue and exits the skin on the side of origin at a comparable short distance from the incision. A rubber or plastic tube or a small roll of gauze sponge is inserted under each loop, external to the skin. The suture is tied to apply tension over the tubing or gauze. A series of such sutures is applied along the incision to distribute tension evenly along the external tubing. The quilled suture may be applied before skin suturing to facilitate accurate positioning of the skin edges.

Near and Far Suture Patterns

Additional tension patterns that may be used to facilitate closure include the far-near, near-far pattern and the far-far, near-near pattern. The suture patterns are applied as their names imply. The first is made

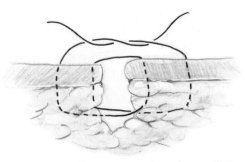

Figure 3–29 Far-near, near-far suture pattern.

by inserting the needle farther from the incision than usual; the needle is then made to pass through the skin and subcutaneous tissue, cross the incision line, and exit through the skin near the incision (Fig. 3–29). The suture is continued across the incision to the side of entrance, where it enters the skin at a point that corresponds (in nearness to the incision) to the point of exit just made on the other side. From the extrance point the suture is passed through the skin and across the subcutaneous incision to exit at a far distance equal to the original. The suture ends are now tied. The advantage of the far-near, near-far suture pattern is that it apposes the skin edges and provides a degree of tension. The disadvantages include excessive amounts of suture material in the area, with double sutures in the incision, and an overlapping suture pattern on the skin. Similar disadvantages and advantages are present with the far-far, near-near suture pattern. In this pattern, the needle is inserted and is passed from a point distant from the skin incision to a similar point on the opposite side, returned across the incision externally, and passed from a point closer to the incision on the original side to a similar close point on the contralateral side (Fig. 3–30). The two ends are then tied.

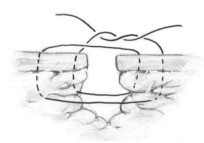

Figure 3–30 Far-far, near-near suture pattern.

Mayo Mattress Sutures

The Mayo mattress suture is an overlapping interrupted mattress pattern. It is useful in midline abdominal closures in large animals and in repair of abdominal hernial defects in all domestic mammals. It is also useful in repair of clefts of the secondary palate. The suture is begun by passing the needle from the outside to the inside of the incision on one side (Fig. 3–31). The needle

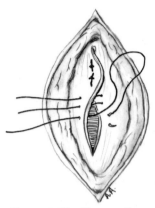

Figure 3–31 Mayo mattress.

is then similarly inserted on the opposite side on the same transverse plane in the same inward direction. It is advanced 0.7 to 1.5 cm and is passed from within to the outside on the second sutured side. Finally, it is returned to the original side and is passed from within to the exterior in the same transverse plane. As the knot is tied, the first area of tissue sutured will overlap the second. A surgeon's knot may be required to overcome distracting forces. Sufficient sutures are placed to close the incision or defect.

Bunnell Sutures

Severed tendons are difficult to appose and maintain in apposition with conventional suture patterns. The suture pattern that is normally recommended for tendon repair is a modified Bunnell (Fig. 3–32A). The suture, usually of nonabsorbable material, is inserted at the cut edge of the tendon and is allowed to cross diagonally to the opposite side of the tendon, where it exits. It is crossed superficially to the side of

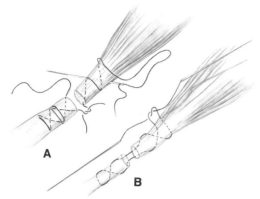

Figure 3–32 Bunnell sutures.

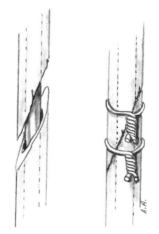

Figure 3–33 Cerclage wiring.

origin and is inserted to pass parallel to the original stitch. On exiting from the tendon it is again crossed superficially and perpendicular to the long axis of the tendon and is introduced on the side of origin. The suture is then inserted retrograde toward the cut edge in a diagonal pattern, passing approximately perpendicular to the previous passages through the tendon, exiting where the first passage exited. It is continued superficially perpendicular to the long axis of the tendon and is reinserted parallel to the previous returning suture. A similar pattern is applied to the opposite tendon end, and the two suture patterns are joined by tying the matching ends of each suture pattern. A double figure X is achieved in each suture that passes through the tendon. Each X is bordered at a point most distal from the cut edge by two perpendicular suture lines that are superficial to the tendon. The Bunnell suture may be shortened to one X pattern if the tendon is short. After alignment, the outer edges of the tendon (tendon sheath) should be apposed with simple interrupted sutures.

An alternate approach would be to use a double-armed suture (Fig. 3–32*B*).

Cerclage and Hemicerclage

Cerclage wiring has been used to appose and fix bone fragments. The term *cerclage* implies that a suture is placed around the bone fragments circumferentially. Cerclage wiring requires strict adherence to the principles of use. Full cerclage is not advisable in short oblique fractures. The length of the fracture should be at least twice the diameter of the bone (Fig. 3–33). Fragments

of bone should be large and readily reducible. One cerclage wire is rarely indicated or successful. No two wires should be placed less than 1 cm apart or less than 5 mm from fracture ends. Wires should be of the same type and large gauge (18 to 20) monofilament. Wires should be applied with a wire tightener (Fig. 1–66) for absolute stability. Wires should be passed through periosteal-fascial attachments as close to the bone as possible; the attachments should be preserved. Slippage in conical bones may be prevented by notching the cortex. Only single loop wires should be applied. Adjacent bones, such as the radius and ulna, should not be incorporated in the same cerclage wire.

Although the previous belief that full cerclage wiring interferes with a presumed longitudinal blood flow has been proved incorrect, some prefer hemicerclage techniques. Several modifications have been described. The first of these modifications consists of passing a wire through a small hole drilled in each bone fragment. The wire passes from one cortex to the medullary canal and exits through the hole in the cortex of the opposite fragment. The wire is then joined externally and twisted (Fig. 3–34). This technique has a tendency to promote rotation of the bone fragments.

The preferred form of hemicerclage wiring is performed by drilling two holes through each bone fragment. A wire is passed through the upper hole in each fragment and run from cortex to medullary canal to cortex. The wire is continued on the surface of the cortex and returned through

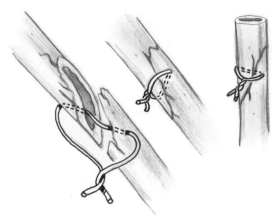

Figure 3–34 Hemicerclage (simplified).

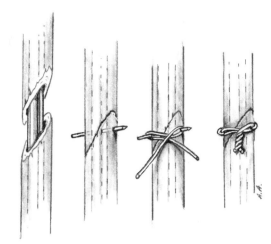

Figure 3–36 Hemicerclage over a Kirschner wire.

the lower hole to pass through the cortex, medullary canal, and cortex in the opposite direction. The ends are then joined and twisted (Fig. 3–35). This form of hemicerclage affords excellent stability.

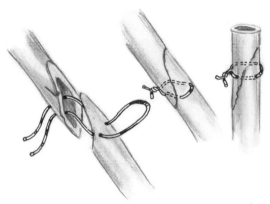

Figure 3–35 Hemicerclage (preferred form).

Hemicerclage may also be applied over a Kirschner wire (Fig. 3–36). In this technique, the bone fragments are aligned and fixed with a Kirschner wire. Monofilament stainless steel wire is placed in a figure-8 around the ends of the Kirschner wire and one side of the bone and is tightened with a wire twister. The wire and pin ends are cut and depressed against the bone to prevent slippage and reduce tissue trauma. Application to Kirschner wires placed through adjacent bone fragments and between stacked intramedullary pins creates a solid fixation. Electrolysis from dissimilar metals is a possibility but has not been observed to date.

USES

The use of specific suture patterns continues to evolve on the basis of clinical experience. Studies of and improvements in suture materials have resulted in a more logical selection of materials for specific needs. Selection of the suture pattern remains in many instances a matter of personal preference. The following suggested uses may serve as a guide based upon the experience of the authors.

Skin

The skin may be adequately apposed with simple interrupted, horizontal mattress, vertical mattress, and continuous apposing or everting sutures. The simple interrupted suture has a tendency to invert when applied to the skin. The surgeon is cautioned against this inversion because it is the one position in which the skin will not heal. Since eversion is preferable, the horizontal mattress suture is the pattern of choice. Continuous suture patterns may be applied in areas where the possibility of self-mutilation is small, as in the thorax or the dorsum of the back. Vertical mattress sutures should be reserved for areas of tension, such as tumor excision and radical mastectomy.

Subcuticular sutures have been used under controlled conditions in the dog and cat for routine surgical procedures. Catgut may be applied as the subcuticular suture material in the dog in order to eliminate the need for suture removal. Many dogs will remove sutures by licking, causing wound dehiscence. Subcuticular sutures may be used following routine surgery if the animal is hospitalized to ensure restriction of activity and to prevent self-mutilation. The added hazard of the subcuticular suture in the dog and cat must be contrasted to the minimum of scarring which results from skin sutures in these animals.

Subcutaneous Tissue

Simple continuous sutures composed of absorbable material are adequate for the closure of subcutaneous tissues in domestic animals. The suture pattern should obliterate all pockets in the tissue, and the knots should be buried.

Fascia

The pattern used in fascia depends on the degree of tension that is apparent. Most incisional planes in fascia are made parallel to the line of tension rather than perpendicular to it. As such, a simple continuous apposition of the fascial plane is adequate. Where fascia is closed perpendicular or at an angle to the line of tension (abdominal midline or paramedian incision), a simple interrupted suture may be used. Where large amounts of fascia have been excised or are absent, a vertical mattress, far-near, near-far, or Mayo mattress pattern may be used.

Peritoneum

The peritoneum of the horse is thin and poorly supports sutures. Muscles are apposed or overlapped using the Mayo mattress pattern. Minimal adhesions develop as the peritoneum proliferates across the incision.

In the dog, the peritoneum is a distinct entity and in all but the caudal abdomen may be sutured in a simple continuous pattern. In the caudal abdomen, a small amount of the muscle superficial to the peritoneum should be incorporated in the pattern to increase holding. A similar small amount of muscle may be incorporated in peritoneal closures in the cat. In the dog

and cat, single layer closure of the peritoneum and muscle fascia in a simple interrupted, through-and-through pattern is generally considered acceptable. Such a pattern should not incorporate large amounts of muscle, for necrosis of that muscle will result. Similarly, the suture pattern must completely close the peritoneum so that small amount of omentum cannot herniate. Although some surgeons prefer a single-layer simple continuous nonabsorbable suture pattern for routine closure of the abdominal peritoneum and fascia, a two-layer closure is preferable; a simple continuous suture should be applied to the peritoneum and a simple interrupted pattern to the external abdominal fascia.

Vessels

Blood vessels, whether venous or arterial, may be closed with simple interrupted or simple continuous suture patterns. The simple interrupted suture is generally used with very small sutures and swaged-on needles and is placed between stay sutures. Blood is allowed to seep through the closure, and the vessel is temporarily occluded or digital pressure is applied until the blood in the incision clots.

Viscera

Considerable debate exists as to the advisability of everting, inverting, or appositional closure of viscera. In the dog, each form appears to allow adequate healing, although more adhesions and microcysts occur when everting closures are used. If properly applied, the direct, appositional, crushing suture provides excellent closure of viscera. For general use in both the bowel and the urinary bladder, a double layer, inverting continuous pattern such as Cushing over Cushing or Cushing over simple continuous is recommended.

Muscle

In small animals, muscles are generally separated rather than cut and do not require sutures. Where a muscle is severed, simple continuous sutures are adequate for apposition. If the muscle is under tension, an alternating horizontal mattress and simple interrupted pattern is advised. Similar patterns may be used in muscle closures in large animals.

Tendons

Tendons are repaired by Bunnell or modified Bunnell closure, with the tendon sheath apposed by means of simple interrupted sutures. Nonabsorbable sutures, particularly wire, are recommended, and the limb should be stabilized in a position without tension on the tendon for at least three weeks.

Bone

When bone fragments are apposed, they should be compressed with a lag screw or cortical screw placed through an overdrilled proximal hole. Such compression of bone fragments facilitates healing. In small fragments, where application of such a compression screw is not possible, hermicerclage wiring with two holes drilled in each bone fragment is recommended. Cerclage wiring, if properly applied, is a logical alternative.

REFERENCES

Abramowitz, H. B. and Butcher, H. R.: Everting and inverting anastomoses. An experimental study of comparative safety. Am. J. Surg., 1971, *121*:52.

Annis, J. R.: Suturing techniques. Proc. A.A.H.A., 1965, 175.

Annis, J. R., and Allen, A. R.: *An Atlas of Canine Surgery*. Philadelphia: Lea & Febiger, 1967.

Annis, J. R., and Allen, A. R.: Intestinal anastomosis. Sm. Anim. Clinic, 1971, *1*:53.

Brunius, V., and Ahren, C.: Healing impairment in skin incisions closed with skin sutures. Acta Chir. Scand., 1969, *135*:369.

Budding, J., and Smith, C. C.: Role of recirculating loops in the management of massive resection of the small intestine. Surg. Gynecol. Obstet., 1967, *125*:243.

Butler, H.: Tendon surgery in small animals. Anim. Hosp., 1966, *2*:236.

Canalis, F., and Ravitch, M. M.: Study of healing of inverting and everting intestinal anastomoses. Surg. Gynecol. Obstet., 1968, *126*:109.

Cohn, I., and Nance, F. C.: Small bowel resection. Surg. Clin. North Am., 1966, *46*:1179.

Cole, W. H.: *Operative Technique in General Surgery*. New York: Appleton-Century-Crofts, Inc., 1955.

Cowley, L. L., and Wall, M.: Comparative strength of single and two-layer open anastomosis of the colon. Am. Surg., 1968, *34*:463.

Cronkite, A. E.: The tensile strength of human tendons. Anat. Rec., 1936, *64*:173.

DeAlmeida, A. D.: A modified single layer suture for use in the gastrointestinal tract. Surg. Gynecol. Obstet., 1971, *132*:895.

Douglas, D. M.: The healing of aponeurotic incisions. Br. J. Surg., 1952, *49*:79.

Forrester, J. C., Zederfeldt, B. H., Hayes, T. L., and Hunt, T. K.: Tape closed and sutured wounds: A comparison by tensiometry and scanning electron microscopy. Br. J. Surg., 1970, 57:729.

Getzen, L. C.: Clinical use of everted intestinal anastomoses. Surg. Gynecol. Obstet., 1969, *128*:1027.

Howard, D. R., Davis, D. G., Merkley, D. F., Krahwin-kel, D. J., Schirmer, R. G., and Brinker, W. O.: Mucoperiosteal flap technique for cleft palate repair in dogs. J. Am. Vet. Med. Assoc., 1974, *165*:352.

Letwin, E., and Williams, H. T. G.: Healing of intestinal anastomoses. Can. J. Surg., 1967, *10*:109.

Loeb, M. J.: Comparative strength of inverted, everted, and end-on intestinal anastomoses. Surg. Gynecol. Obstet., 1967, *125*:301.

Lowenberg, R. I., and Shumacker, H. B., Jr.: Experimental studies in vascular repair. II. Strength of arteries repaired by end-to-end suture, with some notes on growth of anastomoses in young animals. Arch. Surg., 1949, *59*:74.

Markowitz, J., Archibald, J., and Downie, H. G.: *Experimental Surgery*. Baltimore: Williams and Wilkins Co., 1959.

May, G. A., and Andros, G.: A nylon anterior fascial retention suture. Surg. Gynecol. Obstet., 1967, *124*:603.

Mellish, R. W. P.: Inverting or everting sutures for bowel anastomoses: An experimental study. J. Pediatr. Surg., 1966, *1*:260.

Nealon, T. F.: *Fundamental Skills in Surgery*. Philadelphia: W. B. Saunders Co., 1962.

Nelson, P. G., and Dudley, H. A. F.: The tensile strength of small bowel anastomoses in the dog. Aust. J. Surg., 1967, *137*:73.

Partipilo, A. V.: *Surgical Technique*. Philadelphia: Lea & Febiger, 1957.

Piermattei, D. L.: Intestinal anastomosis. Scientif. Proc. 38th Ann. A.A.H.A. Bal Harbour, Fla., April, 1971.

Ravitch, M. M.: Some considerations on the healing of intestinal anastomosis. Surg. Clin. North Am., 1969, *49*:627.

Rhinelander, F. W.: Tibial blood supply in relation to fracture healing. Clin. Orthop., 1974, *105*:34.

Rudy, R. L.: Principles of intramedullary pinning. Vet. Clin. North Am., 1975, *5*:209.

Rusca, J. A., Bornside, G. H., and Cohn, I., Jr.: Everting versus inverting gastrointestinal anastomoses:

Bacterial leakage and anastomotic disruption. Ann. Surg., 1969, *169*:727.

Schwartz, S. I., ed.: *Principles of Surgery.* New York: McGraw-Hill Book Co., 1969.

Smith, R. S.: Management of abdominal incision—a surgery of current practice. Arch. Surg., 1964, 88:515.

Sterner, W.: Surgery of the tendons in dogs. Dtsch. tierarztl. Wochenschr., 1959, *66*:289.

Tauber, R.: *Basic Surgical Skills.* Philadelphia: W. B. Saunders Co., 1955.

Trueblood, H. W., Nelson, T. S., Kohatsu, S., and Oberhelman, H. A., Jr.: Wound healing in the colon: Comparison of inverting and everting closure. Surg., 1969, *65*:919.

Welch, C. S., and Powers S. R., Jr.: *The Essence of Surgery.* Philadelphia: W. B. Saunders Co., 1958.

Wianko, K. B., Kling, S., and MacKenzie, W. C.: Wound healing; Incisions and suturing. Can. Med. Assoc. J., 1961, *84*:254.

Withrow, S. J.: Use and misuse of full cerclage wires in fracture repair. Vet. Clin. North Am., 1978, 8:201.

Withrow, S. J., and Holmberg, D. L.: Use of full cerclage wires in the fixation of eighteen consecutive long bone fractures in small animals. J. Am. Hosp. Assoc., 1977, *13*:735.

Yale, C. E., and VanGemert, J. V.: Healing of inverting and everting intestinal anastomoses in germ-free rats. Surg., 1971, *69*:382.

4

OPERATING ROOM CONDUCT

4

OPERATING ROOM CONDUCT

In the past it was believed by some that animal surgery did not require the strict adherence to aseptic principles found in human surgery. This belief was fostered by incomplete case records, including failure to accurately observe and record postoperative results. Today, the fallacy of this belief is apparent to those who keep accurate records and apply science to surgery. Animal surgery requires the same safeguards from infection as human surgery. The preparation of the surgeon, other operating personnel, patient, observers, equipment, packs, and operating room must follow the rigid routine of accepted operative procedures to insure aseptic surgery. Successful surgery requires thorough knowledge of and strict adherence to aseptic techniques in addition to adequate exposure, hemostasis, gentle tissue handling, and knowledge of anatomy and physiology. Rigid asepsis and gentle atraumatic technique produce a wound that ordinarily heals by first intention.

The principal intent of aseptic surgery is to prevent contamination of the wound inflicted by the surgeon so that the primary goal — healing — will result without infection. The sources of contamination are the patient, the environment (the air, the physical facilities, and so on), the surgical materials and instruments, and the operating room team. Prevention of contamination from these sources requires a routine that demands attention to details and painstaking scrutiny to prevent admission of offending organisms. It necessitates a well-designed surgical suite, adherence to aseptic routine by the operating room team, and a conscientious effort by support personnel in the cleansing of the surgical suite, the sterilization of surgical instruments and materials,

and the proper preparation of the patient. The essential ingredients of every successful operation are simplicity and standardization.

The following discussion presents a method of reducing the chance of contamination from each of the four sources we have named: the patient, the operating room team, the environment, and the instruments. Other methods are available that are equally effective.

PREPARATION OF SURGICAL PACKS

All materials and equipment used in a surgical procedure or entering the operative field must be sterilized. The methods of sterilization are usually classified by the agent used: radiant energy, heat (physical sterilization), chemicals, or gases. Each method varies in its effectiveness and has advantages and disadvantages. Most surgical operations will utilize more than one method of sterilization.

Physical sterilization by moist or dry heat is the most commonly used method of sterilization. Dry heat (baking, flaming) is an effective method of sterilizing sharp instruments because dry heat will not dull edges. However, dry heat sterilization requires one to two hours at a temperature of over 320° F to be effective. The most commonly used method of moist heat sterilization is autoclaving with steam under pressure. It is penetrating, bacteriocidal, and economical. However, autoclaving will dull sharp instruments, scorch fabrics if too dry, may leave packs wet, will not sterilize grease or oils, and will damage some surgical instruments and supplies that are heat labile.

Chemical sterilization was first used by Lister in the 1870s. Chemicals do not dull instruments and are especially useful for smooth, hard-surfaced instruments. They are widely used to wash and disinfect walls and floors. Chemical sterilizing agents are adversely affected by dilution and may be ineffective against spores.

Gases that are used for sterilization are both bacteriocidal and sporicidal. Their penetration and effectiveness at relatively low temperatures make them especially useful for sterilizing surgical supplies made of leather, wool, paper, rayon, plastics, and other heat labile materials. In addition, they sterilize electrical and optical equipment effectively and do not dull instruments. Gases are often flammable and expensive, and they require a long aeration period. Ethylene oxide is a gas commonly used in sterilization.

Instruments and materials must be clean prior to sterilization with any of the agents we have mentioned. Dirt, blood, and other gross contaminants greatly reduce the effectiveness of sterilizing agents. Postoperative cleaning to remove blood can be facilitated by soaking all materials and instruments in cool water and detergent immediately following the surgery. Ultrasonic cleaners are effective for cleaning surfaces of instruments that are otherwise inaccessible (e.g., hinges and clasps). The instruments can then be rinsed and prepared for sterilization. Gowns, drapes, and other fabrics must be laundered.

After drying, the equipment and supplies are arranged for pack preparation. The exact instruments and materials included in a pack will vary with the surgical procedure or with the surgeon's preference. All materials are packed and wrapped to allow opening without contamination.

Pack Preparation for Autoclaving

Autoclaving is the most widely used method of surgical pack preparation. Clean materials, instruments, and supplies to be included in the pack are assembled. The materials are placed in the pack in the order of projected use, with materials used first placed on top. Instruments and materials should not be densely packed; space is required to allow steam circulation within the pack. An excellent precaution is to place a strip of steam-sensitive indicator tape or test culture* in the pack. The former should be placed below the instruments and on the sponges. A good rule is to have available at least twice as many instruments as will be used in the operation. For flexibility, surgical units often have standard packs, packs for special procedures, and additional individually wrapped instruments.

---

* 3M Co., St. Paul, Minn. 55106

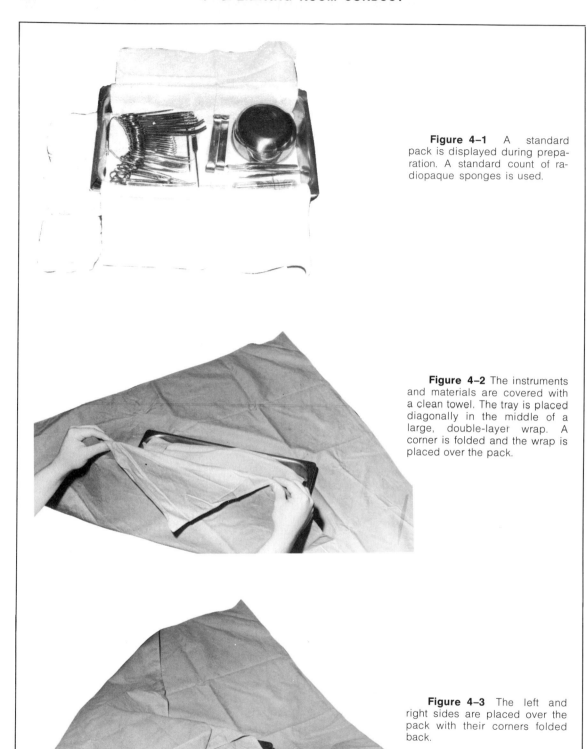

Figure 4–1 A standard pack is displayed during preparation. A standard count of radiopaque sponges is used.

Figure 4–2 The instruments and materials are covered with a clean towel. The tray is placed diagonally in the middle of a large, double-layer wrap. A corner is folded and the wrap is placed over the pack.

Figure 4–3 The left and right sides are placed over the pack with their corners folded back.

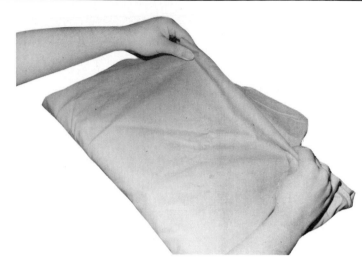

Figure 4–4 The remaining corner of the wrap is placed over the pack and tucked under the two previous folds. The corner remains exposed.

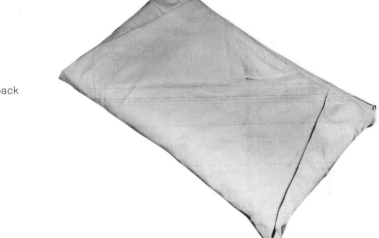

Figure 4–5 The finished pack is compact and tightly folded.

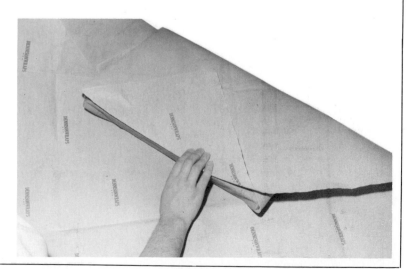

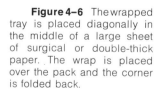

Figure 4–6 The wrapped tray is placed diagonally in the middle of a large sheet of surgical or double-thick paper. The wrap is placed over the pack and the corner is folded back.

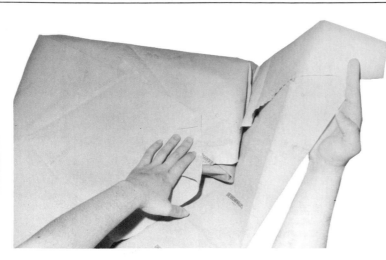

Figure 4-7 The left and right sides of the wrap are placed over the pack and each corner is folded back.

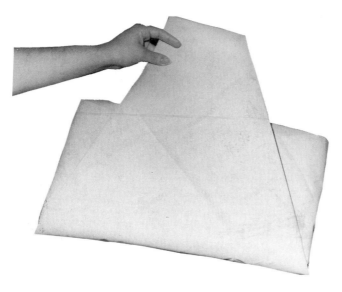

Figure 4–8 The remaining side is placed over the pack and tucked in.

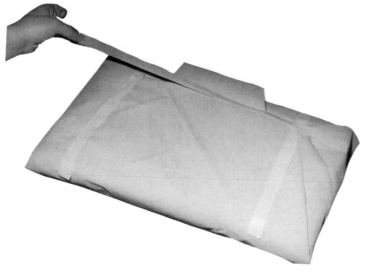

Figure 4–9 The pack is secured with steam-sensitive indicator tape. The end of the tape is turned under for easy removal.

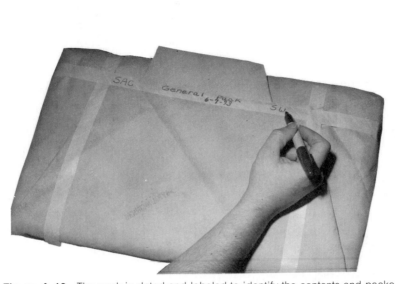

Figure 4–10 The pack is dated and labeled to identify the contents and packer.

Failure in sterilization can result from packs that are too tight or that are improperly loaded in the autoclave. In addition, ineffective equipment, insufficient temperature and pressure, and too short an exposure time may result in sterilization failure. A chart recorder should be used to insure adequate exposure and properly functioning equipment.

Packs should be dry when removed from the autoclave and should be cooled individually on racks. Instrument packs placed on top of each other during cooling may promote condensation of moisture and contamination through wet wrappers. Prompt repair of faulty autoclaves is essential.

Properly wrapped and sterilized packs will remain sterile for up to six months if properly stored. A clean, dry environment is required. If long-term storage is anticipated, the packs should be placed in a plastic bag immediately after autoclaving, and the bag should be heat-sealed. Packs stored in sealed plastic bags remain sterile for up to one year.

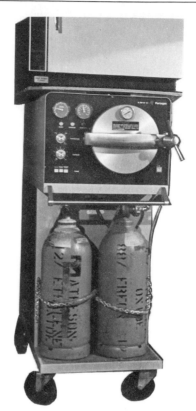

Figure 4–11 Gas sterilization environmental control chamber with commercial aerator on top.

Ethylene Oxide Sterilization

Ethylene oxide is a highly penetrating gas that is quite effective in the sterilization of surgical equipment.

Ethylene oxide sterilization may be obtained in a chamber with environmental control (Fig. 4–11). In the unit shown,* two time-temperature cycles are available. The gas is exhausted to the outside or to a water drain. Similar sterilization at less cost may be obtained with canisters or trays and an ethylene oxide vial (Fig. 4–12). The wrapped instruments are placed in a plastic bag.** The vial of ethylene oxide is broken and placed in the plastic bag and the bag is sealed. The canister is covered and timing is begun. After sterilization, wrapped and unwrapped equipment should be aerated by shelf storage for one day or by treatment in a commercial aerator (top, Fig. 4–11).†

---

*AMSCO Portagas Sterilizer, American Sterilizer Co., P.O. Box 92078, Chicago, IL 60690
**Anprolene Sterilizer, H. W. Anderson, Inc., Oyster Bay, NY 11771
†Steri-Vac Aeration Cabinet 33, 3 M Company, St. Paul, MN 55101

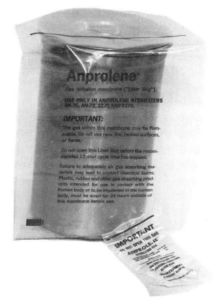

Figure 4–12 Gas sterilization canister with gas diffusion membrane bag.

Pack Preparation for Ethylene Oxide Sterilization

Preparation of materials for gas sterilization is relatively easy.

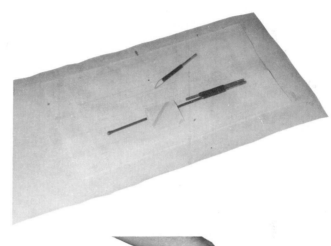

Figure 4-13 Clean materials or instruments are placed in a tube of polyethylene or in plastic with paper backing.

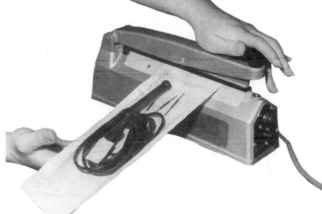

Figure 4–14 The ends are doubly sealed. A sealing iron or steam-sensitive indicator tape can be used. If a sealing iron is used, a piece of indicator tape is placed in the pack. Sterilization tubing may be purchased with indicator banding.

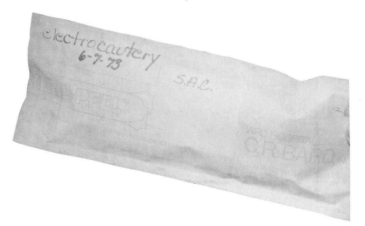

Figure 4–15 The backing sheet or indicator tape is dated. Contents should be labeled for easy recognition. Gas instruments in packets sealed with indicator tape remain sterile for approximately six months. Those that are heat-sealed remain sterile for up to one year.

PREPARATION OF THE OPERATIVE SITE

The decision to submit a patient to surgery should not be made without adequate medical evaluation of the condition of the animal. In this way — provided there is due consideration given to the inherent risks of the surgical procedure — an accurate prediction of results can be made. Food should be withheld from the patient for at least six hours prior to surgery; water should be allowed. A bath is recommended the day prior to surgery, especially in the case of heavily soiled animals. If possible, the animal should be exercised within an hour of anesthesia to encourage voiding. If the patient fails to void, the bladder can be expressed while the animal is under anesthesia. It is good surgical practice to place and maintain an intravenous catheter throughout the surgical procedure. In addition, a heated water pad covered by another pad or a towel should be placed on the table prior to positioning the patient, in order to decrease hypothermia during surgery.

Disagreement exists concerning the best routine and agents to use in the preparation of the surgical site. However, a consensus has been reached that the initial preparation, clipping, and scrubbing should take place outside the surgical suite and that the routine must be accomplished gently.

Preparation of the surgical site includes the following:

1. Removal of hair.
2. Cleansing with a surgical scrub and warm water to remove dirt and water insoluble materials.
3. Use of a scrub with residual antibacterial activity so that flora rising to the surface will be inhibited.
4. Application of an effective germicide. Ideally, the vehicle should be a fat solvent for greater skin penetration.

The germicide may be applied to sterile sponges placed over the surgical site. The sponges are removed after transport to the surgical site. Germicide may be reapplied. If contamination in transit is suspected, the site should be rescrubbed and the germicide applied. Bacteriologic studies have shown the necessity of a germicidal agent. They have also established that an antiseptic applied as a spray is less effective than the same agent applied with friction. After application, the germicide should not be wiped off but should be allowed to dry on the surgical site. The germicide requires approximately four minutes to achieve a maximal effect. The best skin germicide — the agent against which all others must be compared — remains 1 per cent iodine in 70 per cent ethyl alcohol (by weight) applied with friction. Iodine tincture should not be applied to the scrotum.

Tamed iodophor solutions may be applied as a final germicide rinse but should be wiped with alcohol before surgery. Alcohol (70 per cent) is considered by many an adequate germicidal rinse. The germicidal agent should be applied in a circular pattern from the incision to the periphery, as is done in the preparatory scrubbings.

PREPARATION OF THE SURGEON AND OPERATING ROOM CONDUCT

Members of the surgical team, observers, and operating room personnel are potential sources of direct or indirect patient contamination. Policies on attire and operating room conduct should be established and enforced. All persons entering the operating suite, whether an operation is in progress or not, should be appropriately clothed. In addition, the individual should be clean and should observe good habits of personal hygiene and grooming. Observation gowns and disposable shoe covers can be worn over the street clothes of observers and others entering the surgical suite.

Caps and masks are necessary whether an operation is in progress or not. Three types of caps are shown in Figure 4–25. The cap must completely cover the hair of both the head and face, and the mask must cover both the mouth and nostrils. The mask is secured by shaping the top edge reinforcement snugly about the nose. Disposable masks are the most effective filters of exhaled air and are less likely to become wet. Disposable caps and masks should not be reused. Cloth caps and masks must be laundered after each use. Fogging of glasses can be prevented by polishing them with ordinary soap.

Text continued on page 84

Preparation of the Operative Site
The Small Animal

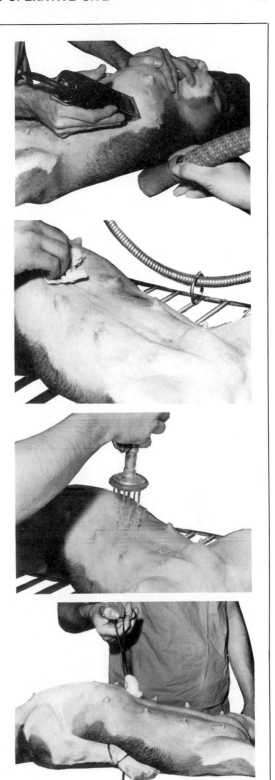

Figure 4–16 A generous area surrounding the proposed incision site is clipped with a number 40 clipper blade. Removed hair is vacuumed to reduce contamination. In some cases it appears advisable to remove all hair from the incision site by shaving or utilizing a depilatory agent. The irritation these procedures cause to the skin must be weighed against the small amount of hair left by the clipper blade. Abrasions caused by shaving become heavily colonized with organisms.

Figure 4–17 The surgical site and surrounding area are cleansed with a surgical scrubbing agent that is active, non-irritating, and will not inhibit skin healing. The site is wetted and the scrub agent is applied with a sterile cotton swab or surgical sponge, not a brush. A limited amount of water is utilized. The two most commonly used surgical scrub agents are povidone-iodine* and hexachlorophene.† Several bacteriological comparisons of these agents have produced conflicting data. A 1970 review article recommended PVP-iodine for surgical site preparation and hand cleansing. The authors concur in this recommendation.

Figure 4–18 Following the first scrub, the area is rinsed. At least two similar scrubs follow, with a residue from the last scrub left on the patient while it is transported into the surgical suite. The surgical area should be scrubbed in a circular pattern, starting at the incision site and moving outward. When the periphery is reached, the sponge is discarded, and the scrubbing agent is wiped away with clean, sterile sponges.

Figure 4–19 A germicidal solution is applied by sterile sponge. The patient is transported to the surgical suite and positioned, and the germicidal agent reapplied.

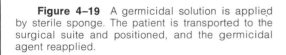

*Povidone-iodine is sold under the name Betadine by the Purdue Frederick Co., Norwalk, Connecticut.

†Hexachlorophene is sold under the name pHisoHex by Winthrop Laboratories, New York, New York.

Preparation of the Operative Site

The Large Animal

Preparing the large animal patient for surgery requires following the same sound practice of preparation as described for the small animal. Previous grooming, such as thorough brushing and wiping the coat and cleaning the feet, should be carried out before anesthesia induction. Excessive amounts of rinse water should be avoided to keep the surrounding hair and floor dry.

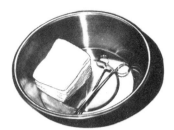

Figure 4–20　　Typical scrub tray consists of a sterile bowl, sponge forceps, and gauze sponges. This is used for the final scrub.

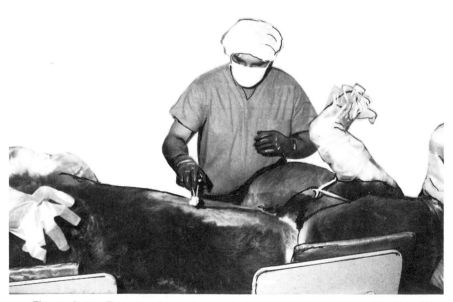

Figure 4–21 The gloved operator starts the scrub at the proposed incision line. All four feet are placed in plastic disposable obstetrical sleeves. The penis is tied out of the way.

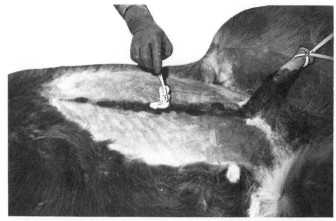

Figure 4–22 The final prep is started at the proposed incision site and is scrubbed out from that point.

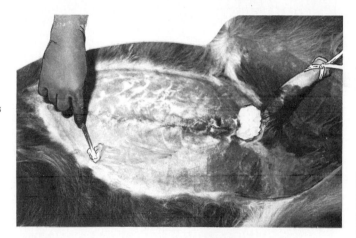

Figure 4–23 The periphery is scrubbed after the incision site.

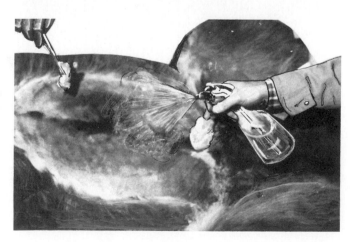

Figure 4–24 An antiseptic spray is applied to the scrubbed area, starting at the center and working out to the periphery. Excessive spray should be avoided to prevent the solution from running across the incision line.

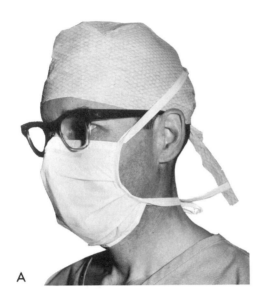

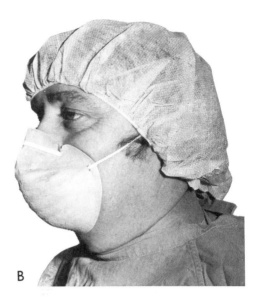

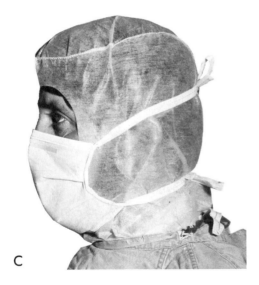

Figure 4–25 The standard cap is acceptable for short hair (A). Other caps cover long hair (B), and hoods are used for side burns and beards (C).

The surgeon and other members of the surgical team should wear a scrub suit or special clothes, shoes worn only in the surgical area or shoe covers, and cap and mask.

The conventional operating room attire is a short-sleeved cotton shirt and long pants or a similar easily washed dress.

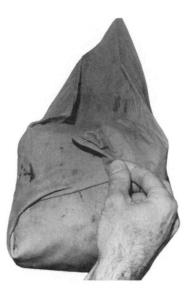

Figure 4–26 Prior to scrubbing, the surgeon and other members of the operating team open their gowning packs. These packs usually include the surgical gown and hand towel. The pack is opened by removing the indicator tape and unfolding the corners. The pack is placed so that the first corner is folded away from the individual opening the pack.

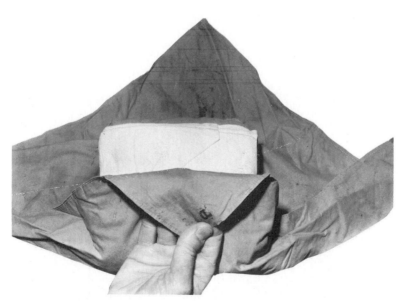

Figure 4–27 In opening the pack, only the folded back edges of the corner are grasped. Thus, the wrap shields the towel and gown from the hand.

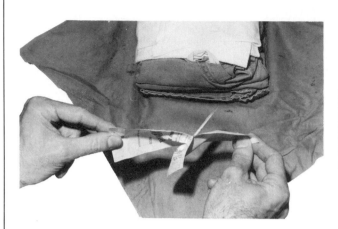

Figure 4–28 A package of sterile gloving cream is placed on the sterile wrap next to the gown and towel. This is accomplished by pulling back the edges of the wrapper and dropping the sterile cream onto the wrap. In placing the gloving cream, the hands do not violate the air space above the sterile materials.

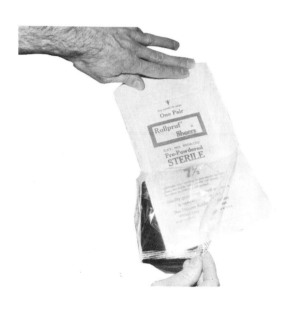

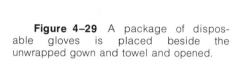

Figure 4–29 A package of disposable gloves is placed beside the unwrapped gown and towel and opened.

Some surgical units use non-disposable gloves. These require cleaning, checking for punctures during powdering, packaging, and autoclaving. Cost analysis indicates that disposable gloves are more economical. In addition, there is less danger of contamination from a defective glove. If operating room personnel are available, an assistant opens the gowning and supply packs as the surgeon scrubs.

A deep sink with facilities that permit the adjustment of water flow without touching the faucets is used for scrubbing. A knee or foot control is preferred. Warm water should be used for scrubbing. A timing clock set prior to scrubbing is helpful. The surgical scrubbing agents of current preference are povidone-iodine and hexachlorophene. Iodophor scrub solutions (with detergent) are three times more effective than hexachlorophene preparations at maintaining low bacterial counts for at least two hours following scrubbing.

Considerable controversy surrounds what constitutes a complete scrub. It can be measured by time or by brush strokes per surface. The time and number of strokes may vary, depending on the frequency of scrubs and previous environmental contacts. Whatever the case, the objective of the scrubbing process is to reach and thoroughly cleanse all the skin area of the hands and forearms. Scrubbing times of three to 15 minutes or five to 20 brush strokes per surface have been advocated. However, both factors — vigorous scrubbing and exposure time — are important. The current preference is for either a five minute surgical scrub or 10 brush strokes per surface,

with at least two thorough scrubs and rinses.

The hands are held higher than the elbows during scrubbing, rinsing, and drying to prevent contamination from water dripping or running from the upper arm (an unsterile surface) onto the forearms and hands. In addition, caution should be taken to avoid unnecessary wetting of the scrub suit.

Text continued on page 100

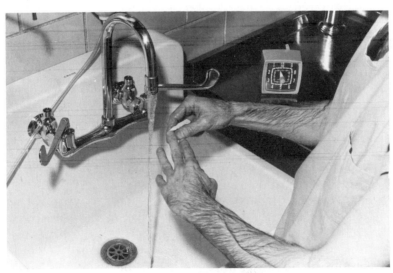

Figure 4–30 The fingernails should be trimmed to 1 mm or less and cleaned with a disposable nail cleaner.

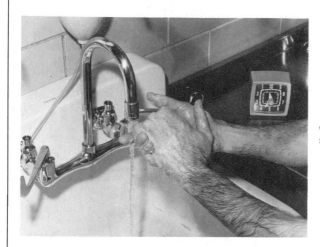

Figure 4–31 The hands and forearms are washed for 30 to 60 seconds with the surgical scrub.

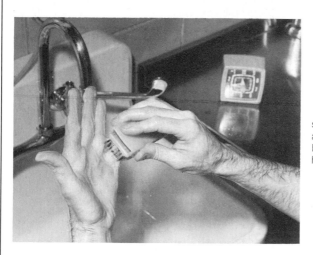

Figure 4–32 The hands are methodically scrubbed with a sterile brush, scrubbing agent, and water. Each surface of each finger should be scrubbed, as well as the surfaces of the hands and arms.

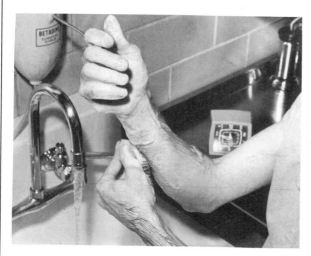

Figure 4–33 The process is repeated on the opposite arm, with care being taken to scrub all surfaces with the brush.

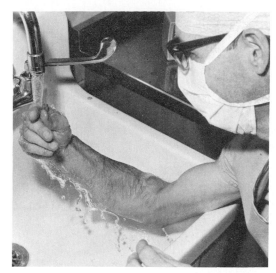

Figure 4–34 Both arms are rinsed and re-scrubbed.

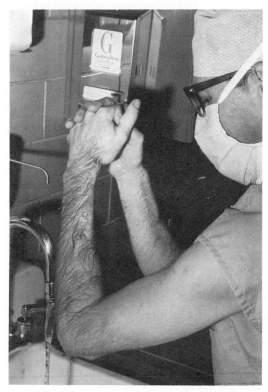

Figure 4–35 When the scrub is complete, the hands and arms are rerinsed with the hands still held above the elbows.

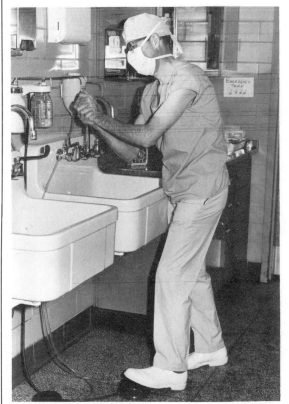

Figure 4–36 The application of a germicide to the hands and forearms following scrubbing reduces the bacterial flora and the chance of surgical contamination. The germicide can be applied by basin dip, spray, or dispenser. However, it is most effective when the hands and forearms are massaged as it is applied. Since up to 50 per cent of surgical gloves contain holes subsequent to a surgical procedure, the value of this practice is apparent.

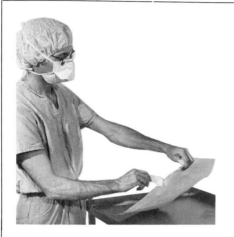

GOWNING AND GLOVING

Disposable Gown

Figure 4–37   An easy-open tab is removed to expose the wrapped gown and towel.

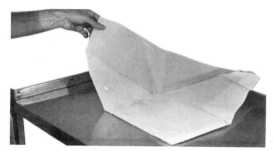

Figure 4–38   The sterile gown and towel wrap are opened without passing the hands above the opened pack. The pack is opened before scrubbing or by an assistant as the surgeon scrubs.

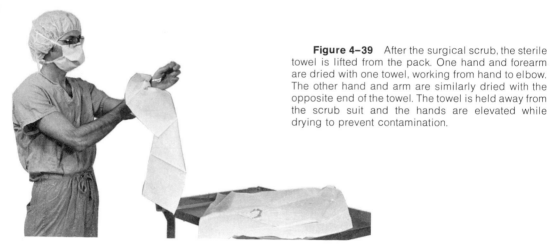

Figure 4–39   After the surgical scrub, the sterile towel is lifted from the pack. One hand and forearm are dried with one towel, working from hand to elbow. The other hand and arm are similarly dried with the opposite end of the towel. The towel is held away from the scrub suit and the hands are elevated while drying to prevent contamination.

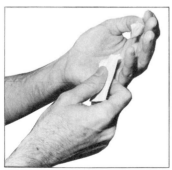

Figure 4–40   Sterile gloving cream is applied and massaged on the hands for equal distribution.

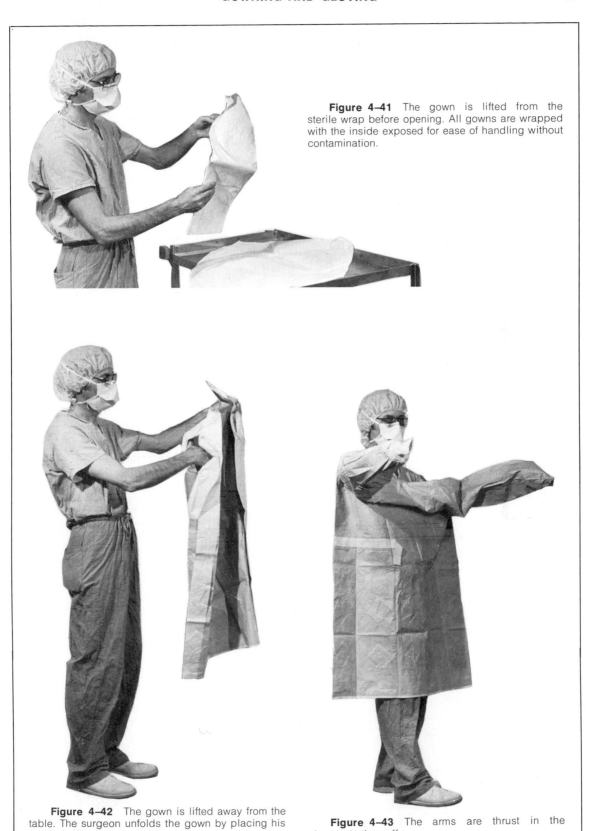

Figure 4–41 The gown is lifted from the sterile wrap before opening. All gowns are wrapped with the inside exposed for ease of handling without contamination.

Figure 4–42 The gown is lifted away from the table. The surgeon unfolds the gown by placing his hands in the appropriate arm holes.

Figure 4–43 The arms are thrust in the sleeves to the cuff.

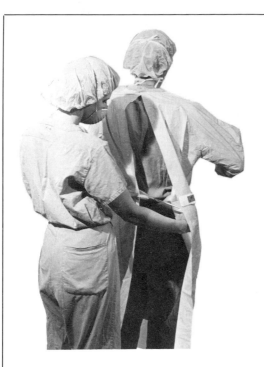

Figure 4–44   An assistant closes the neck fastener and ties the inside waist tie.

Closed Gloving

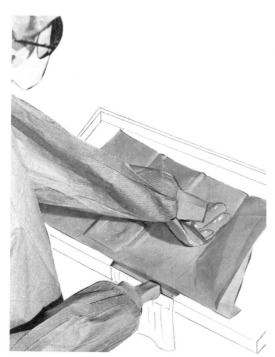

Figure 4–45   The right glove is lifted from the previously opened glove pack with the covered left hand.

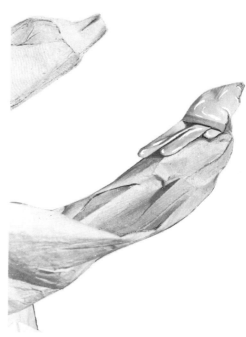

Figure 4–46   The right glove is placed on the covered right hand with the fingers toward the elbow and the thumb toward the surgeon's right thumb. The edge of the cuff is grasped with the thumb and fingers by the sleeve-covered right hand.

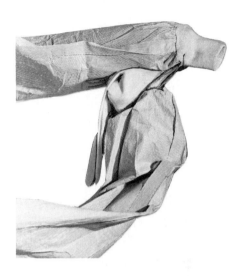

Figure 4–47 The cuff is grasped with the covered left hand and is folded over the cuff of the right sleeve.

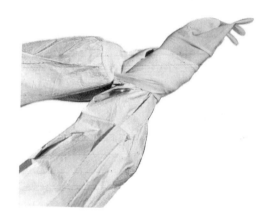

Figure 4–48 The cuff of the glove and sleeve are pulled toward the surgeon as the fingers enter the glove.

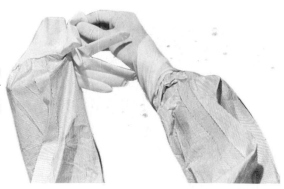

Figure 4–49 The left glove is lifted and placed cuff-to-cuff with the fingers toward the surgeon and the thumb toward the surgeon's thumb. The cuff is grasped with the covered left thumb and fingers.

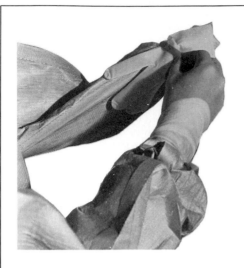

Figure 4–50 The remaining glove cuff is pulled over the end of the cuff of the gown.

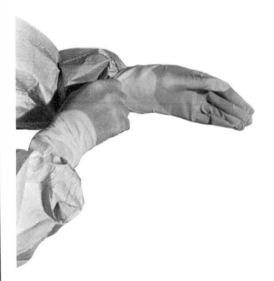

Figure 4–51 The cuff of the glove and the gown are pulled toward the surgeon as the fingers and thumb are inserted into the left glove.

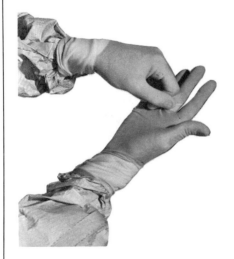

Figure 4–52 The gloves are adjusted for comfort.

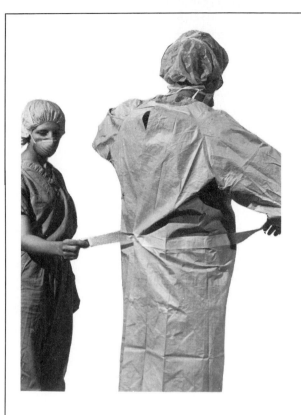

Figure 4-53 The Kendall gown is equipped with a sterile right front tie, which the surgeon grasps. An assistant grasps the tab covering the expansive back tie.

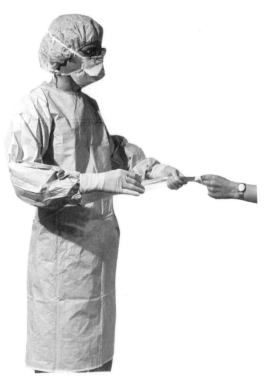

Figure 4-54 The assistant pulls the back tie around the surgeon's left side until he grasps it and then pulls the covering tab away.

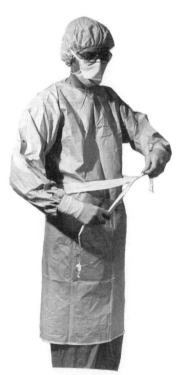

Figure 4-55 The surgeon ties the right and back ties to complete gowning.

Cloth Gown

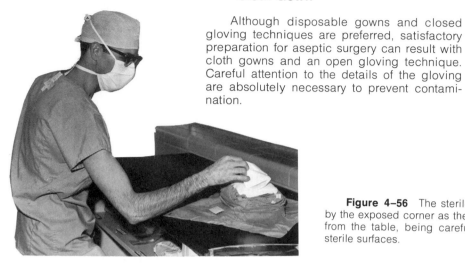

Although disposable gowns and closed gloving techniques are preferred, satisfactory preparation for aseptic surgery can result with cloth gowns and an open gloving technique. Careful attention to the details of the gloving are absolutely necessary to prevent contamination.

Figure 4–56 The sterile towel is lifted by the exposed corner as the surgeon steps from the table, being careful to avoid unsterile surfaces.

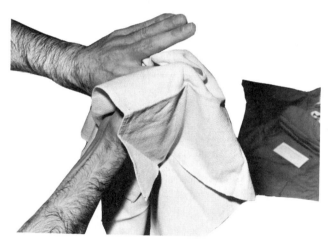

Figure 4–57 One hand and forearm are dried with one towel end. Care is exercised to carefully dry between the fingers and to avoid contaminating the other end of the towel against the scrub suit. The forearm is dried with a circular motion proceeding from the wrist to the elbow.

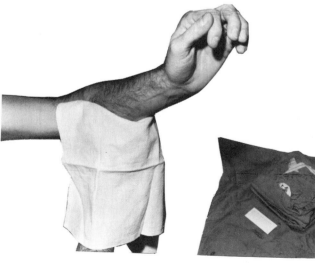

Figure 4–58 The other hand and forearm are similarly dried with the opposite towel end. Contamination may easily occur during the drying process owing to careless control of the sterile towel.

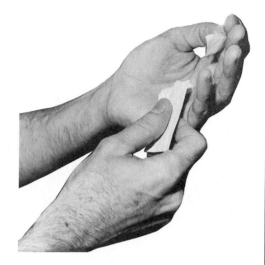

Figure 4–59　The sterile gloving cream packet is opened and the cream is expressed on the hands. The hands are massaged with the cream for equal distribution.

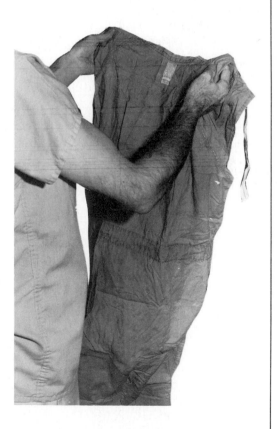

Figure 4–60　Surgical gowns are folded with only the inside exposed. The gown is lifted away from the table, and the surgeon allows it to fall open by grasping it at the top with the inner surface facing him.

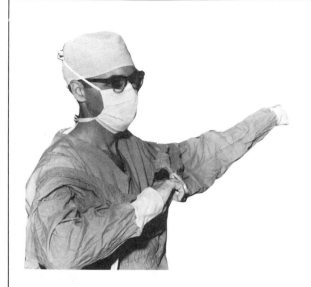

Figure 4–61   The arms are inserted into the arm holes without touching the outer surface. Assistance is preferable while gowning; however, with care it is possible to self-gown without contamination. In the illustration, the surgeon is pulling his arms into the gown by grasping the top tie. The tie must be placed over the shoulder or tied if handled.

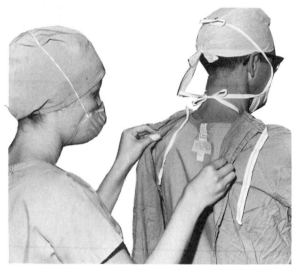

Figure 4–62   The gown may be pulled on by an assistant touching only the inner surface.

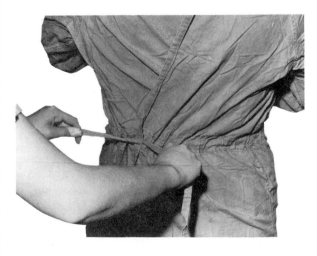

Figure 4–63   The gown is tied at the neck and snugly secured at the waist by the assistant or, in self-gowning, by the surgeon.

Open Gloving

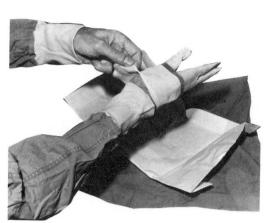

Figure 4–64 One of the gloves is lifted from the opened gloving container by its turned-down cuff. The glove is pulled on the hand with a rotating motion. Neither the gown nor the outer surface of the glove is touched.

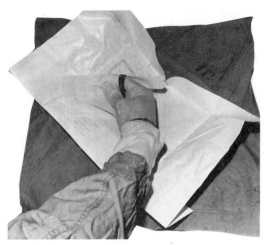

Figure 4–65 The opposite glove is lifted by placing the gloved fingers into the cuff.

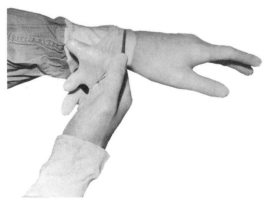

Figure 4–66 With the gloved fingers under the cuff, the glove is placed on the ungloved hand. The folded cuff protects the gloved hand from contamination. It is pulled over the cuff of the gown following insertion of the hand.

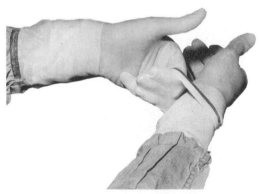

Figure 4–67 The fingers are slipped under the cuff of the first glove to be donned so as to lift the glove cuff over the gown cuff.

OPENING PACKS

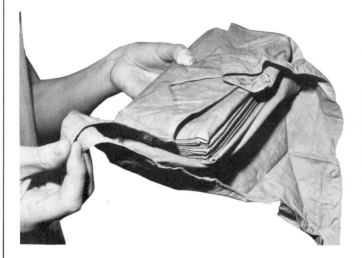

Figure 4–68 Assistants open the sterile packs without touching their inner surfaces and present them to the surgeon. This can be done by removing the indicator tape and unfolding one corner at a time. If assistance is not available, the surgeon must open the packs and materials prior to scrubbing.

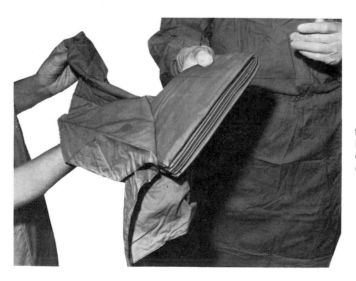

Figure 4–69 The surgeon grasps the sterile drapes, pulling them toward his body while the assistant carries the outer wrap down and away. The wrap covers the hand of the assistant.

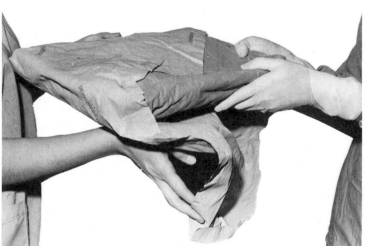

Figure 4–70 Instrument trays are similarly presented, with the assistant carefully removing the paper wrap as the surgeon grasps the sterile cloth wrap. The surgeon places it on the instrument stand and opens it using the wrap as an instrument stand cover.

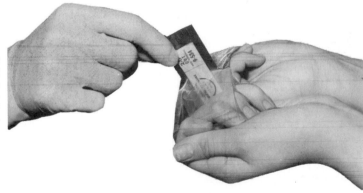

Figure 4–71 Sterile packs of suture material are presented by pulling apart the flaps of the outer wrapper. This prevents contamination of either the surgeon or the contents of the sterile package.

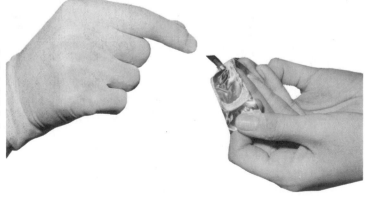

Figure 4–72 In a similar manner the assistant opens sterile blades and other required instruments and supplies. A mosquito forceps may be used to grasp small items. Transfer forceps may be used by an assistant to retrieve supplies.

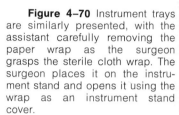

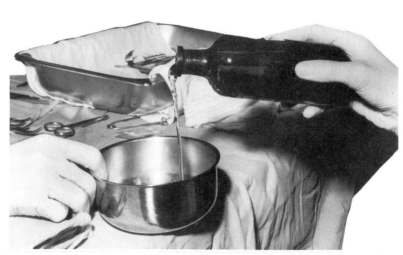

Figure 4–73 The assistant fills the bowl with sterile saline. The surgeon holds the bowl away from the sterile instrument stand. At no time is an unsterile item or instrument allowed to pass over the sterile field. The instruments should be arranged on the instrument stand to facilitate easy access during the surgical procedure.

PRECAUTIONS TO MAINTAIN STERILITY

In attaining and maintaining a sterile field, sterile surfaces must touch sterile articles only, and unsterile articles must contact unsterile surfaces only. Violation of this principle results in contamination and possible infection. The following additional precautions should be observed to aid in maintaining a sterile field.

1. Members of the operating team never turn their backs on a sterile surface.

2. An unsterile area should not be touched or leaned over.

3. Sterile instruments should never fall below the edge of the surgical table.

4. Arms and hands should remain above the waist and below the shoulder. The front of the surgical gown between the waist and shoulder is the area considered sterile.

5. When receiving instruments or materials, lift them up. Do not drag them over the edges of their containers.

6. Keep all sterile surfaces dry. Moisture may cause contamination of a sterile field. Place the saline bowl in the instrument pan.

7. Avoid excessive movement during surgery (e.g., arm waving or traffic in and out of the operating suite).

8. Avoid shaking of gowns, towels, drapes, and other materials; let them fall open by gravity. Shaking increases air currents and the possibility of contamination.

9. Keep conversation in the operating suite to a minimum during surgery. It has been shown that bacterial contamination of the operating room atmosphere increases proportionately with the amount of conversation.

10. Never fold your arms; clasp them in front of the body above the waist.

If this routine is carefully executed, a sterile field in which the instruments and the surgeon are wholly uncontaminated will be established at the start of the surgical procedure.

SURGERY ROOM CLEANLINESS

The careful preparation of the patient, surgeon, and operating supplies will be wasted if the surgical environment is contaminated. Lister recognized this in 1865 when he advocated the use of carbolic acid spray to disinfect the operating room. Scrupulous postoperative clean-up as well as specific daily and weekly cleansing routines must be established to limit contamination. Ideally, cleaning should be done by trained housekeeping personnel, but whoever is charged with the responsibility should have well-planned routines that are meticulously performed.

DAILY CLEANING. Damp dusting of all flat surfaces, lights, and other operating room furniture is a routine practice. It is carried out approximately one hour before scheduled incision time in order to remove particles of dust that may have settled in the room during the inactive period. A clean cloth dampened with a germicidal solution or alcohol is used. The room itself should be neat and free of unnecessary operative equipment. Following surgery, areas contaminated by organic debris such as blood should be cleaned with a detergent and a disinfectant, e.g., quaternary ammonia compounds, chlorhexidine, or iodophores. A cup of vinegar in the solution will neutralize detergent resistant residues.

All floors and soiled areas of the surgical suite must be cleaned with a disinfectant. Wet vacuuming is the method of choice for floor care in the operating suite. However, mops are still in fairly wide use despite the overwhelming evidence against their effectiveness in reducing contamination. If a wet mop must be used, a double bucket technique should be employed. All mops are laundered daily or soaked in fresh germicidal detergent solution for 20 minutes. At no time should a dry mop be used in the operating room. The recommended technique of wet vacuuming requires that the operating room floor be flooded with a disinfectant released from an automatic spraying device or from a pump sprayer like those used on gardens. Areas of soiling should be wiped, and more disinfectant should be added. The disinfectant is then picked up with a vacuum cleaner. Kick buckets and other waste receptacles should be carefully cleansed and disinfected. Disposable plastic liners may be used and disposed of after each surgical procedure to facilitate cleaning. Special effort should go into cleaning the scrub sinks and soap dispensers; it is essential to remove oily film residues left by scrub detergents. Other areas of the operating room and storage equipment should be spot-cleaned daily. Mechanical friction should always be included in the cleansing disinfection process.

WEEKLY CLEANING. The walls and ceilings should be wiped down with a germicidal cleaning solution weekly. Cabinets and other operating room equipment should be cleansed. The exterior of air conditioning grills should be vacuumed and filters should be changed as needed.

In choosing and utilizing disinfectants, it is important to remember that their effectiveness is drastically reduced in the presence of organic materials. Thus, surfaces should be first cleansed with a good detergent and flushed with clean water. In the case of heavily soiled areas, additional disinfectant should be applied to the area following initial cleansing. Disinfection is not an instantaneous process. The rate and efficiency will depend on the available concentration of the disinfectant, the duration of contact, and the number of organisms present. The agent selected for disinfection should be effective against a wide range of pathogens, including spores, non-toxic to the tissues of animals and man, non-corrosive to steel, aluminum, or plastics, and economical. The most commonly used disinfectants are quaternary ammonia compounds, chlorhexidine, and iodophores.

In addition to thorough cleaning, routine monthly sampling utilizing Rodac plates* or swab cultures is recommended in the operating suite.

---

*Available from Bio Quest, Division of Becton Dickinson and Co. P. O. Box 243, Cockeysville, Md. 21030.

REFERENCES

Berman, Richard E., et al.: Evaluation of hand antisepsis. Arch. Environ. Health, 1969, Vol. 18.

Cole, W., et al.: Inadequacies of present methods of skin preparation. Arch. Surg., 1964, 89:215.

Crowder, Virgil H., et al.: Bacteriological comparisons of hexachlorophene polyvinylpyrrolidone-iodine surgical scrub soaps. Am. Surg., 1967, 33:11.

Dineen, P. L.: An evaluation of the duration of the surgical scrub. Surg. Gynecol. Obstet., 1969, 129:1181–1184.

Dineen, P. L.: Clinical research in skin disinfection. A.O.R.N.J., 1971, 14:73–78.

Dodson, Thomas, et al.: A study of various surgical scrubs by glove counts. Surg. Gynecol. Obstet., 1967, 124:57.

Eitzen, H. E., Ritter, M. A., French, M. L., et al.: A microbiologic in-use comparison of surgical handwashing agents. J. Bone Joint Surg. (Am.), 1979, 61:703–406.

Fitzgerald, R. H., Jr., and Washington, J. A., II: Contamination of the operative wound. Orthop. Clin. North Am., 1975, 6:1105–1114.

Handler, Seymour: Preoperative preparation of the skin. Minn. Med., 1921, 54.

King, Thomas, C., et al.: Skin degerming practices: Chaos and confusion. Am. J. Surg., 1965, 109:695–698.

Kowalski, J. J., et al.: Is your disinfection practice effective? J.A.A.H.A., 1973, Vol. 9.

Laufman, H., et al.: Scanning electron microscopy of moist bacterial strike-through of surgical materials. Surg. Gynecol. Obset. 1980, 150:165–170.

Lowbury, E. J. L., and Lilly, H. A.: Use of 4% chlorhexidine detergent solution (Hibiscrub) and other methods of skin disinfection. Br. Med. J., 1973, 1:510.

Markowitz, J., Archibald, J., and Downie, H. G.: Experimental Surgery, 5th ed. Baltimore, Md.: Williams and Wilkins, Co., 1964.

Moylan, J. A., and Kennedy, B. V.: The importance of gown and drape barriers in the prevention of wound infection. Surg. Gynecol. Obstet., 1980, 151:465–470.

Nealon, T. F.: Fundamental Skills in Surgery, 2nd ed. Philadelphia: W. B. Saunders Co., 1971.

Paul, J. W.: Efficacy of a chlorhexidine surgical scrub compared to that of hexachlorophene and povidine-iodine. VM/SAC, May, 1978, 573–579.

Peers, J. G.: Clean-up techniques in the operating room. Arch. Surg., 1973, 107:596–599.

Perkins, E. W.: Aseptic Technique for Operating Room Personnel, 2nd ed. Philadelphia: W. B. Saunders Co., 1964.

Printup, R. H.: Surgery cleaning procedures. Executive Housekeeping, 1972, 6:74–80.

Prioleau, W. F.: A safe method of drying hands and forearms after the surgical scrub. Am. J. Surg., 1967, 113:586–587.

Raahave, D.: Effect of plastic skin and wound drapes on the density of bacteria in operation wounds. Br. J. Surg., 1976, 63:421–426.

Richards, R. C.: Surgical skin preparation. Proc. AAHA, 1972, 630–635.

Smith, R. M., and Young, J. A.: Simplified gas sterilization. A new answer for an old problem. Br. J. Anaesth., 1968, 40:909–914.

Subcommittee on Aseptic Methods: Report to the Medical Research Council on Aseptic Methods in the Operating Suite. Lancet, 1968, 1:705–759, 763–768, 831–839.

Wangensteen, O. H., et al.: Surgical cleanliness, hospital salubrity and surgical statistics, historically considered. Surgery, 1972, 71:477–493.

White, J. J., et al.: Skin disinfection. Johns Hopkins Med. J., 1970, 126:169–176.

White, J. J., and Duncan, A.: The comparative effects of iodophor and hexachlorophene surgical scrub solutions. Surg. Gynecol. Obstet. 1972, 135:890–892.

5

WOUND DRESSING

5

WOUND DRESSING

BANDAGING MATERIALS

The variety and quality of material used for bandaging animals has improved in recent years. These improvements have added to the armamentarium of the surgeon. The essential and classically reliable materials are always abundantly available; diverse improved forms have made bandaging considerably easier for the clinician.

Sponges

Sponge is a woven fabic (usually cotton) that is porous and folded into a square or rectangular shape. Sponges are available in sizes ranging from $2'' \times 2''$ to $8'' \times 10''$ (or larger); the latter size is used for rectangular abdominal packs. Sponges filled with a cellulose absorbent material may be purchased. Some sponges are marked with a radiopaque line. Sponges used in bandaging should be sterile. They may be purchased individually sterilized or may be sterilized with steam or ethylene oxide in groups.

Gauze

Gauze is woven fabric packaged in rolls from one to six inches wide and of variable length. Relatively inexpensive and available in white or camouflage colors, it has served as the basic material for bandaging in medicine for many years. It may be purchased sterile or may be autoclaved. The disadvantage of gauze is that it is not pliable and tends to buckle unless purposely turned 180° at the point of rotation.

Elastic Gauze

Several new forms of elastic gauze are available. These are marketed under names such as Kling,* Coban,† and Vetrap.‡ The latter two have the expansible material Lycra incorporated in them so that they are pliable and apply some pressure. The elasticity is beneficial but can cause stricture in a limb if it is not applied judiciously. Elastic gauzes and bandage materials tend to adhere to themselves; therefore, minimal external taping is required to fix the material firmly in place. Because they do not adhere to the skin or hair, there is no discomfort in removal.

Adhesive Tape

The quality of adhesive tape has improved. Most available adhesive tape is porous, a feature that permits air access to the underlying gauze and wound and frees the wound from the detrimental effects of entrapment of moisture. Modern adhesive tapes are less likely to deteriorate under adverse temperature and storage conditions than were their predecessors. Elastic adhesive tapes are available that permit the application of a mild degree of pressure while maintaining the other qualities of adhesive materials (Elastikon§).

---

*Kling elastic gauze is manufactured by the Johnson and Johnson Co., New Brunswick, N.J.
†Coban elastic gauze is manufactured by the 3M Co., St. Paul, Minn.
‡Vetrap elastic gauze is manufactured by the 3M Co., St. Paul, Minn.
§Elastikon Porous Adhesive Tape is manufactured by the Johnson and Johnson Co., New Brunswick, N.J.

Other Materials

The standard dressing materials — gauze, tape, elastic gauze, and sponges — are supplemented by many other products. Both gauze and gauze sponges that have been impregnated with petrolatum or antimicrobial ointments and sterilized are available. Non-stick bandages have gained popularity. The gauze is fixed to tape on the outer surface but is structured to prevent adherence to the wound. Non-stick bandages tend to trap moisture.

Abdominal pads* absorb moisture from the wound. When changed regularly they are an excellent adjunct to draining wounds. Sponge rubber materials of various sizes have been designed to facilitate the use of the metal shoe or other splint materials by eliminating adherence to the underlying tissue and by absorbing excessive pressures. Combine Roll† is a double-layer gauze with absorbent cotton interspersed within the material. This gauze and cotton sandwich provides a thick padding material which, because of the outside gauze, is strong.

A similar dressing may be fabricated by folding roll absorbent cotton in gauze or cheesecloth. It is totally satisfactory when applied full width but loses its composition when cut. Two forms of roller padding are available for splints: Sof-Roll,‡ which is smooth, and Specialist Cast Padding,§ which is corrugated. These products provide excellent padding for all types of splints. Stockinettes‖ is a woven cloth that may be applied under cast padding prior to plaster application (Chap. 8) or may be doubled and used (sterile) as covering for the skin in orthopedic procedures (Chaps. 1 and 7). Stockinette is also used in bandaging the body, head, and neck and is available in 100 per cent and cotton-polyester blends.

Absorbent cotton may be purchased in several grades, with the highest quality recommended for general bandaging. In lower grades, cotton strands tend to separate and cause uneven thickness under the bandage. The relatively high cost of top-quality absorbent cotton is worth bearing. Sponge rubber, foam rubber, and other materials have been bonded to an adhesive base for application and direct attachment to the skin. Such materials have found limited utilization in veterinary medicine, but their use may increase with time. Stabilization of erect ears in dogs with these materials appears promising but is difficult to maintain without external tape. Moisture is trapped when the foam is encased in tape. Doughnut-shaped bandages are useful on pressure points to prevent and treat decubital ulcers. The standard butterfly and adhesive bandages commerically available for small wounds in humans have found limited application in animals because of their relatively poor holding ability without additional fixation. Similarly, non-allergenic tapes have been fabricated at various materials and may eventually find additional usage in animals.

Bandages are used to prevent wound contamination, seromas, and self-mutilation. Their usefulness in the prevention of wound contamination is generally short-lived, rarely in excess of 24 to 36 hours. Under aseptic conditions wounds heal quite satisfactorily without bandage. A large number of bandages that tend to obliterate minor tissue spaces are used to prevent seroma formation. Such bandaging is recommended in animals, both postoperatively and in the presence of other trauma. These bandages are generally removed within four to five days. The cardinal rule is to avoid a pressure ring and pressure points. Evenly applied pressure from the foot proximally is not detrimental. A ring bandage may cause extreme edema, even to the point of skin seepage within 24 hours, and gangrene of the limb peripheral to the bandage. Ring bandages should be avoided whenever possible. Bandages help to prevent self-mutilation in animals despite the fact that they may be readily removed by manipulation with teeth or unpadded claws. The bandage at least tends to forewarn the clinician that the animal is worrying the wound and allows other measures to be taken. One such measure, the use of the side brace, will be described in this chapter. Other forms of collars are commercially available that have a use in both the dog and the cat for the prevention of self-mutilation.

*Kendall Co., Boston, Mass.
†Combine Roll is manufactured by Johnson and Johnson, New Brunswick, N.J.
‡Sof-Roll is manufactured by Johnson and Johnson, New Brunswick, N.J.
§Specialist Cast Padding is manufactured by Johnson and Johnson, New Brunswick, N.J.
‖Orthopedic Stockinette is manufactured by Johnson and Johnson, New Brunswick, N.J.

BANDAGING THE TRUNK

Gauze and Tape

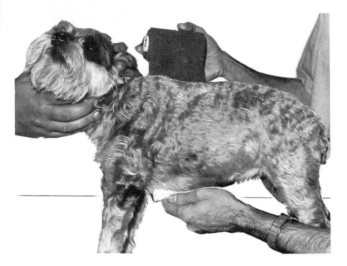

Figure 5–1 A sterile sponge is placed over the incision and elastic gauze (Vetrap) rolled around the trunk.

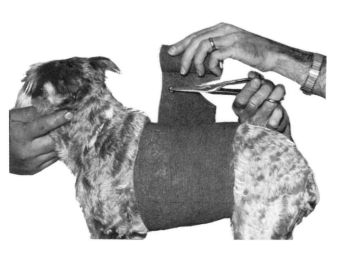

Figure 5–2 The gauze is applied to cover the abdomen and part of the chest, preventing slippage from the chest to the abdomen.

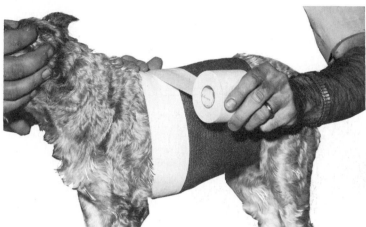

Figure 5–3 The gauze bandage is covered with adhesive tape, which is attached to the skin cranial and caudal to the gauze.

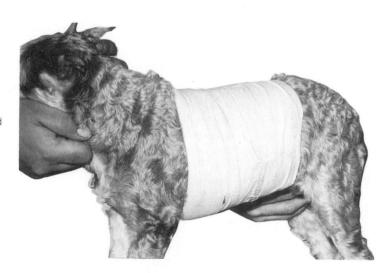

Figure 5–4 The finished gauze and tape bandage.

Stockinette Bandage of the Trunk

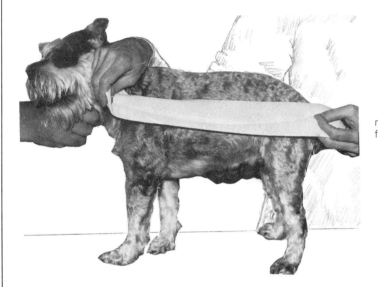

Figure 5–5 Stockinette is measured in comparable length from a suitable diameter roll.

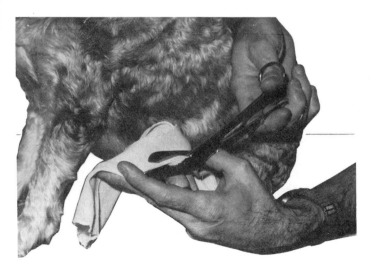

Figure 5–6 Two holes are cut on the proposed ventral surface for placement of the limbs. The distance between the holes should be approximately one-third the circumference of the stockinette.

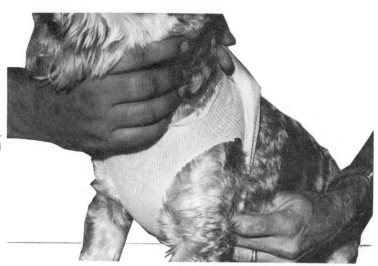

Figure 5–7 The stockinette is placed over the head and forelimbs.

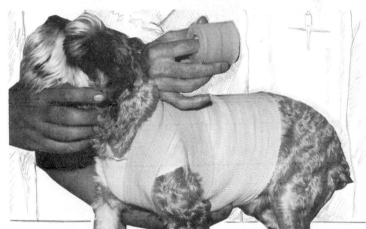

Figure 5–8 Sterile gauze is placed over the incision beneath the stockinette, and the stockinette is taped with elastic tape.

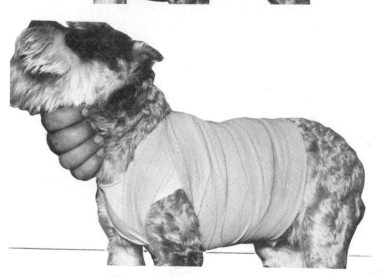

Figure 5–9 The tape is allowed to adhere to the skin or hair at the cranial and caudal edges of the bandage.

The Inguinal Region — Gauze

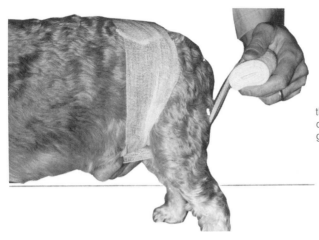

Figure 5–10 Gauze is applied to circle the abdomen in the region of the flank and continued from the right flank through the inguinal region to the left perineal area.

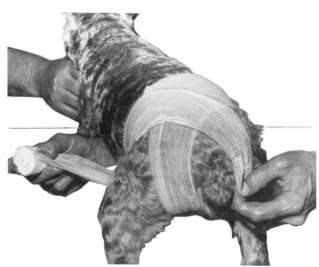

Figure 5–11 The gauze encircles the trunk again and continues across the right perineal region, through the inguinal area, to the left flank.

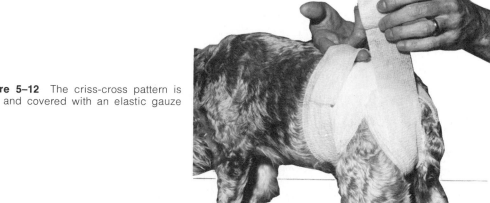

Figure 5–12 The criss-cross pattern is repeated and covered with an elastic gauze wrap.

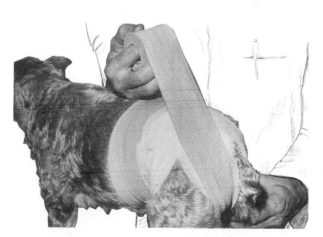

Figure 5–13 Elastic tape is applied in a similar fashion and attached to the skin at the cranial edge of the bandage.

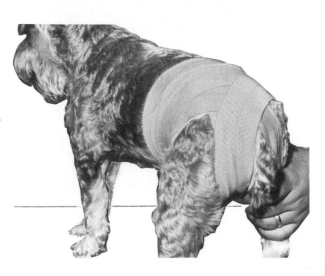

Figure 5–14 The criss-cross pattern of the bandage allows free limb motion with minimal pressure on the peripheral veins and free exposure of the vulva and anus.

The Inguinal Region — Stockinette

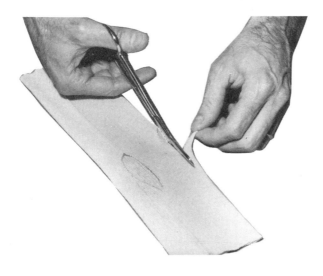

Figure 5–15 Two elliptical holes are cut approximately one-third the circumference of the stockinette apart.

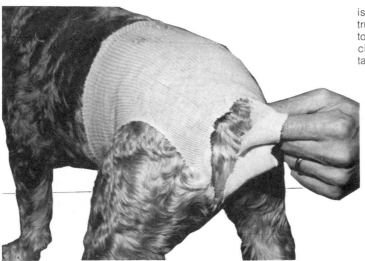

Figure 5–16 The stockinette is placed over the rear limbs and trunk; the excess stockinette caudal to the tail and perineal region is excised with scissors to expose the tail, anus, and vulva.

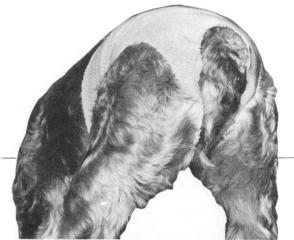

Figure 5–17 To prevent accumulation of urine and feces in the bandage, the exposure should be ample.

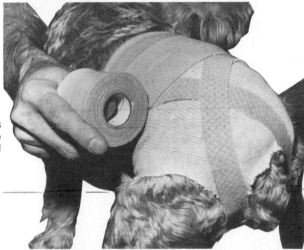

Figure 5–18 One-inch elastic tape is criss-crossed to cover the stockinette in the perineal and inguinal regions and covered cranially with two-inch elastic tape.

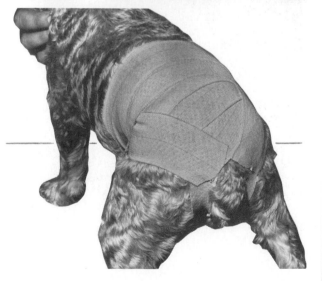

Figure 5–19 Additional pieces of elastic tape may be applied to create even pressure throughout the inguinal bandage.

BANDAGING THE HEAD

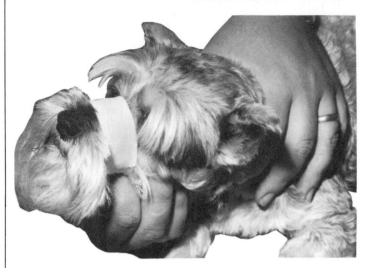

Muzzle

Figure 5–20 Standard adhesive tape placed firmly around the muzzle will provide sufficient support for selected mandibular fractures and temporomandibular luxations. The bandage, which should be tight enough to ensure apposition of the canine teeth, will be sufficiently loose in 12 to 24 hours for the tongue to be protruded. Obstruction of the trachea is a hazard should vomiting occur with the muzzle in place. A pair of bandage scissors should be readily available.

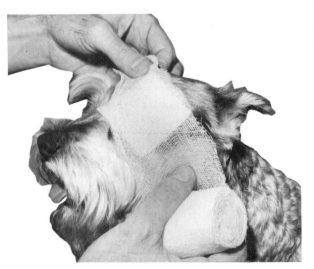

The Eye

Figure 5–21 A sterile 2″ × 2″ gauze bandage is applied over the eye and secured with elastic gauze applied from the dorsal surface of the head across the bandage to below the ear.

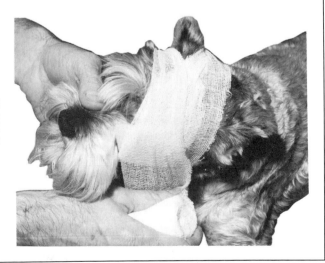

Figure 5–22 The bandage is continued below the head and caudal to the opposite ear. The bandage is alternated cranially and caudally to the ear opposite the eye being bandaged.

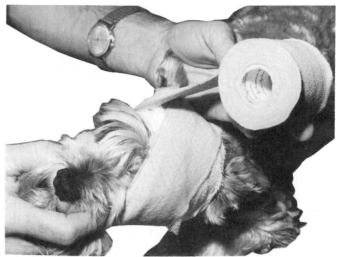

Figure 5–23 The gauze is covered with elastic tape in a similar fashion with fixation cranial and caudal´to the opposite ear.

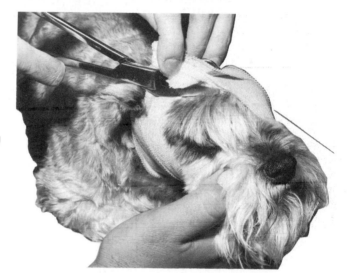

Figure 5–24 Excess bandaging is removed dorsal to the opposite eye.

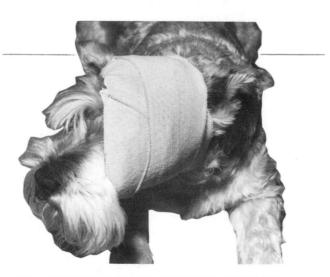

Figure 5–25 The bandaged eye is well protected by a padded elastic bandage offering minimal pressure in the cervical region and adequate exposure for the opposite, unbandaged eye.

Ear — Erect

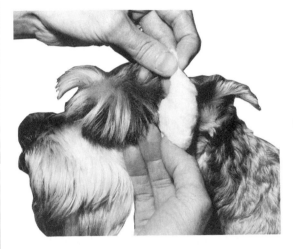

Figure 5–31 An absorbent cotton cone is wound to approximate the shape of the external ear.

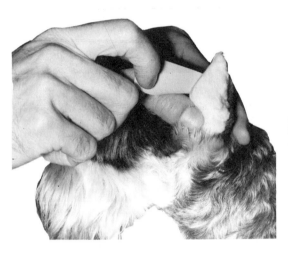

Figure 5–32 The cone is placed in the ear canal, and a strip of adhesive tape is applied from the craniomedial surface across the cotton to the caudal surface of the ear.

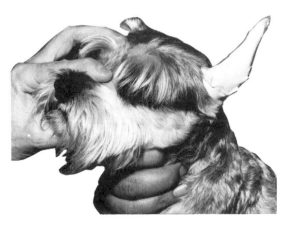

Figure 5–33 Four short strips of tape are similarly applied around the ear and the enclosed cotton cone.

Ear — Variations

Many techniques have been used to support ears after cropping. In one, the ears are pulled medially over the head and are taped to each other. In others, the ears are taped individually or together. Several of these are illustrated here. None exceeds the value of taping around a core of cotton, in the author's opinion.

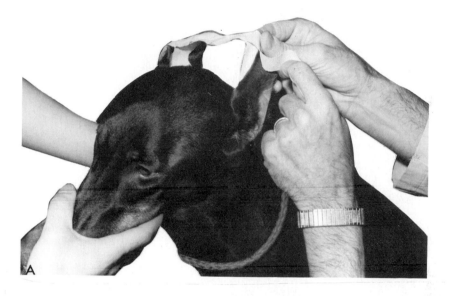

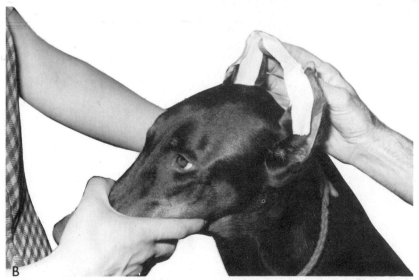

Figure 5–34   Adhesive tape strips are applied to the medial and lateral surfaces of the leading edge of each ear. The strips are continuous and are joined between the ear tips.

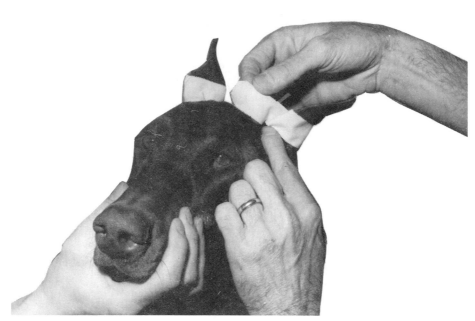

Figure 5–35 A single piece of 1 inch tape is applied to the proximal third of each ear, turning the leading edge medially and forming a cone of the ear.

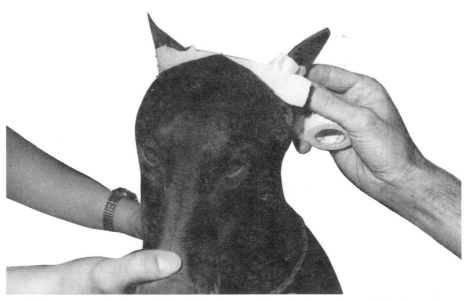

Figure 5–36 A piece of adhesive tape may be added on the cranial edge to keep the ears erect.

The Neck

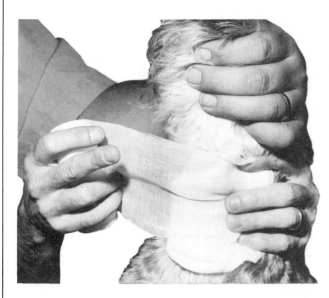

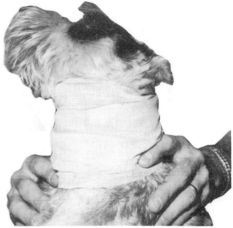

Figure 5–37 The neck is bandaged with a simple cerclage bandage applied over a sterile cotton pad.

Figure 5–38 The gauze should be applied smoothly and with minimal tension.

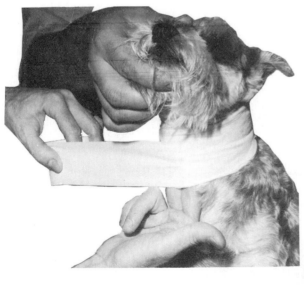

Figure 5–39 The gauze is covered with adhesive tape but should freely admit two fingers at each end between the bandage and the neck.

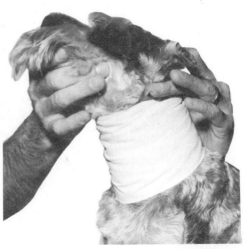

Figure 5–40 The finished bandage affords stability with minimal pressure on the vessels and trachea.

BANDAGING THE EXTREMITIES

The Limbs

Standard Gauze Bandage

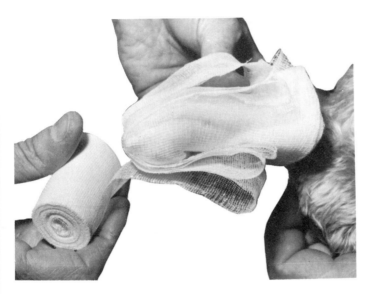

Figure 5–41 The foot is covered with a sterile 4″ × 4″ sponge, and layers of gauze are reflected to cover the distal extremity.

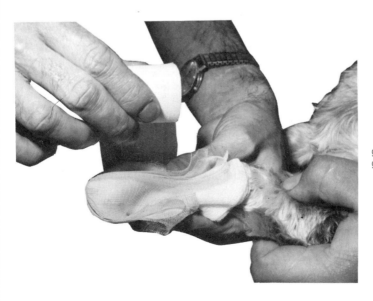

Figure 5–42 The layers of gauze are covered with a wrap of gauze roll.

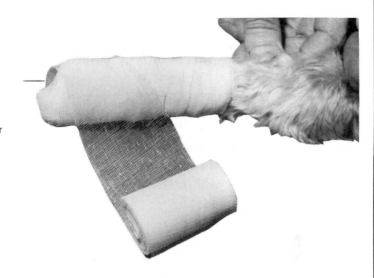

Figure 5–43 A second layer is applied from proximal to distal.

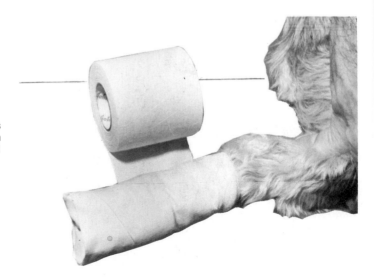

Figure 5–44 The bandage is covered with adhesive tape from the distal extremity to the proximal hair.

Post Bandage

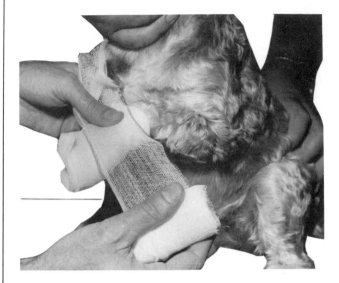

Figure 5–45 A sterile 4″ × 4″ sponge is covered on the lateral surface with elastic gauze, the end of which is free.

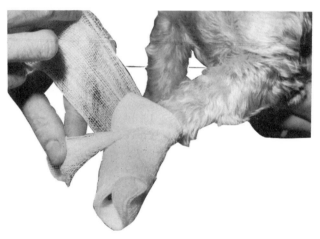

Figure 5–46 The gauze is circled around the foot proximal and distal to the free end.

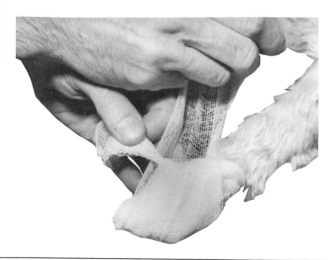

Figure 5–47 The pattern is repeated to cover the proximal bandage and the distal end of the foot.

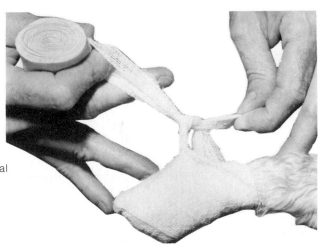

Figure 5–48 The proximal and distal ends of the gauze are tied.

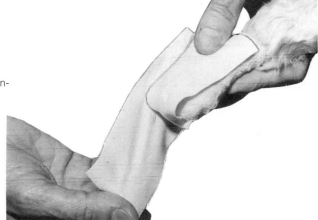

Figure 5–49 The distal end of the bandage is covered with tape.

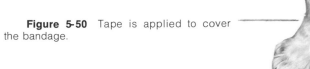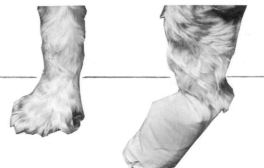

Figure 5-50 Tape is applied to cover the bandage.

*Tubegauz**

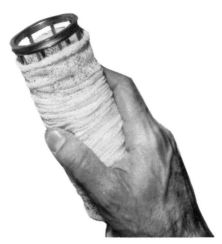

Figure 5–51   A thin, stockinette-like gauze tube may be used to bandage a limb. The gauze (Tubegauz*) is applied from a bale and covers a sterile sponge.

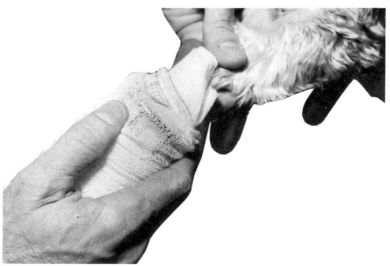

Figure 5–52   The unrolling is begun at the distal third of the proposed bandage site, with the bale being rotated on its long axis to apply greater or lesser tension to the bandaging material.

---

*Tubegauz is a product of the Scholl Manufacturing Co., Inc., Chicago, Ill.

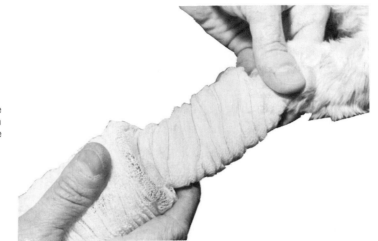

Figure 5–53 The bandage is applied proximally and then distally to the distal end of the foot.

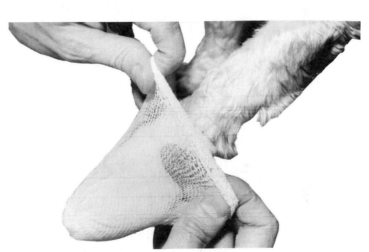

Figure 5–54 The tube of gauze is severed several inches distal to the foot and is reflected over the bandage.

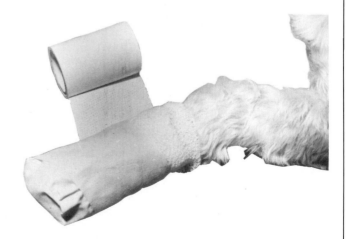

Figure 5–55 Tape is applied to the distal end of the bandage and is then wound circumferentially over the bandage and skin or hair proximal to the bandage.

Modified Robert Jones

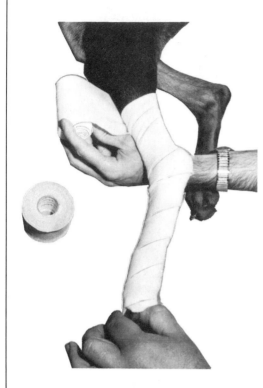

Figure 5–56 Cast padding is applied to the limb from the foot proximally to the mid-femoral or mid-humeral region.

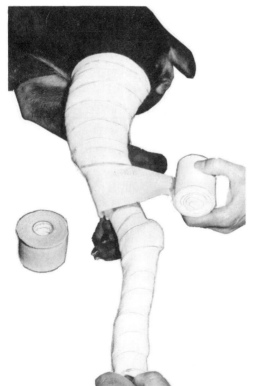

Figure 5–57 The cast padding is applied in an overlapping, smooth pattern.

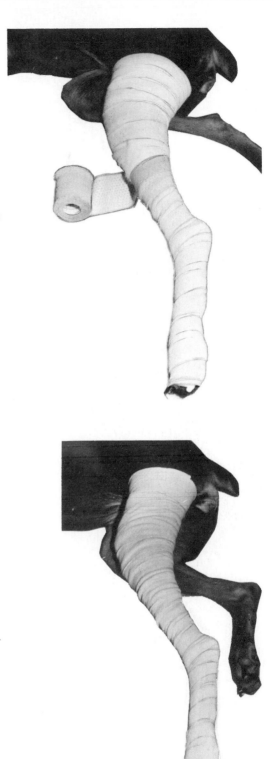

Figure 5–58 The cast padding is covered with elastic tape applied from the foot proximally.

Figure 5–59 Elastic tape may be fixed to the hair or skin.

Bergh Bandage

An excellent modification of the limb bandage was developed by Dr. Robinson and two surgical technicians at Henry Bergh Memorial Hospital of the ASPCA, New York, NY. Although proposed for cats, the modifications·is equally useful in short-limbed dogs. Use of one or two longitudinal fixation tapes will improve the holding quality of a modified Robert Jones bandage in any small animal.

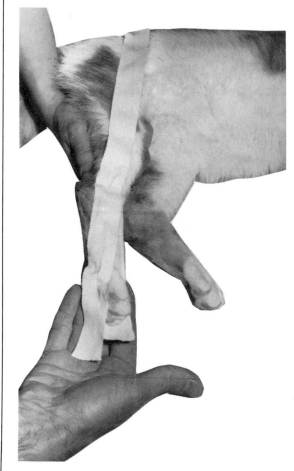

Figure 5–60 A longitudinal strip of adhesive tape is placed on the lateral and medial side of the limb, avoiding wounds.

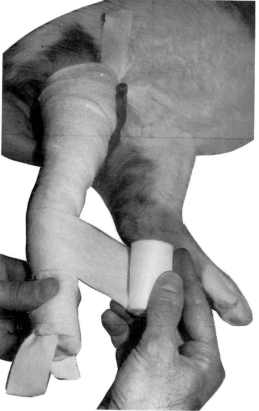

Figure 5–61 The wound is dressed and padded with cotton, then wrapped with elastic gauze.

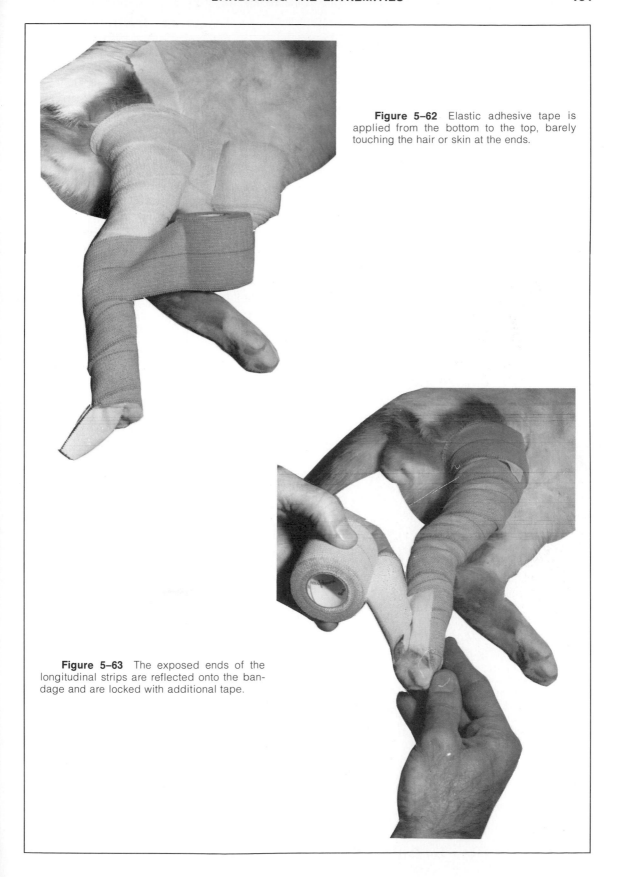

Figure 5–62 Elastic adhesive tape is applied from the bottom to the top, barely touching the hair or skin at the ends.

Figure 5–63 The exposed ends of the longitudinal strips are reflected onto the bandage and are locked with additional tape.

The Hip — Standard

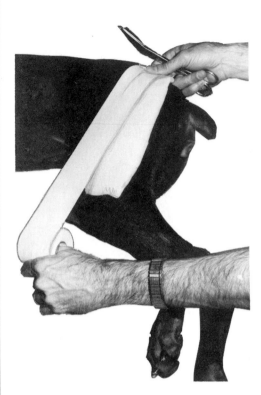

Figure 5–64 Sterile sponges are applied over the incision site.

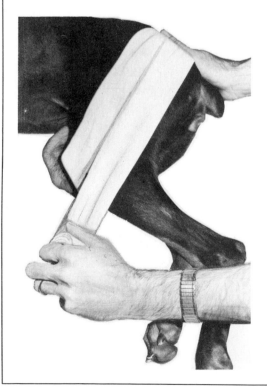

Figure 5–65 Adhesive tape is placed caudal, cranial, and lateral to the sterile sponges.

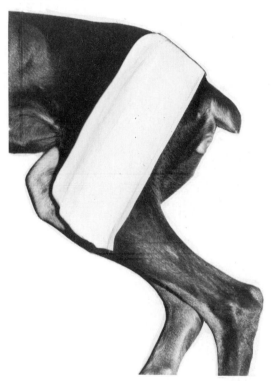

Figure 5–66 The adhesive tape should converge dorsal to the hip and reflect cranial and medial to the stifle.

The Hip — Padded

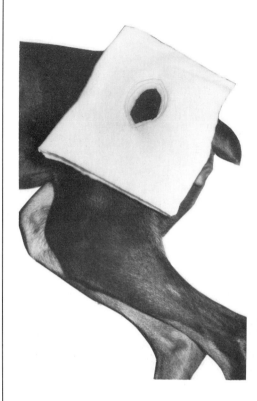

Figure 5–67 A hole is cut in the center of a double layer of Combine Roll or similar padding material.

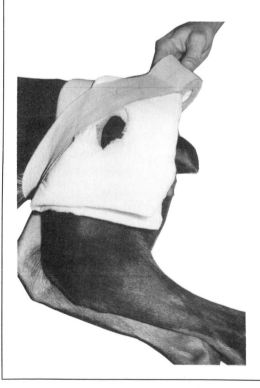

Figure 5–68 The Combine Roll is fixed to the limb with elastic tape.

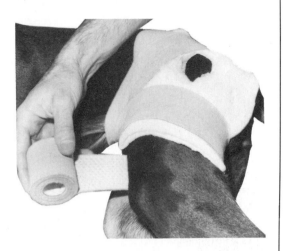

Figure 5–69 The elastic tape circles the flank and upper thigh region.

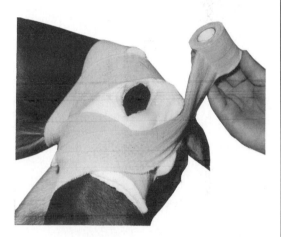

Figure 5–70 The padded bandage is useful in the prevention and treatment of decubital ulcers.

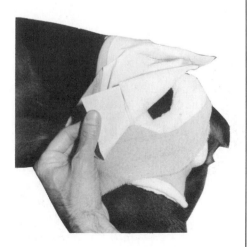

Figure 5–71 Sterile or medicated sponges may be applied to the skin.

The Shoulder

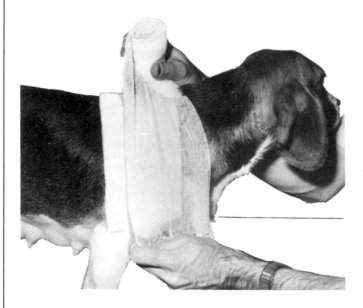

Figure 5–72 A sterile sponge is applied over the incision.

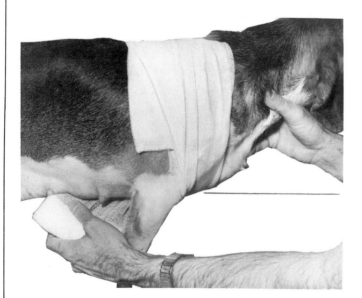

Figure 5–73 The sponge is covered with roll gauze circling the body.

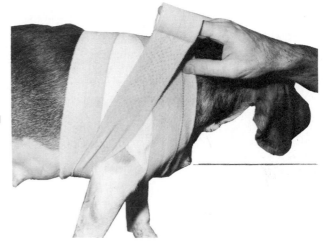

Figure 5–74 Elastic tape is applied to the gauze.

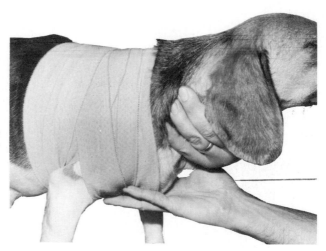

Figure 5–75 The tape encircles the trunk, passing cranial and caudal to the opposite limb.

The Tail

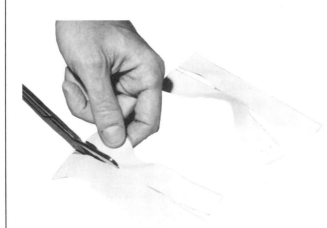

Figure 5–76 Two strips of tape are cut on their proximal and distal ends to make many-tailed tapes.

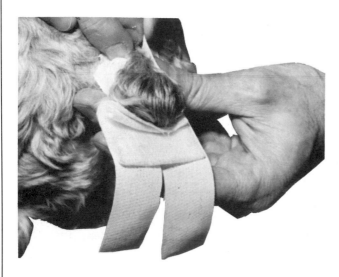

Figure 5–77 One strip of tape is applied over a small, sterile sponge, and the proximal ends are reflected on the lateral sides of the tail so that they overlap.

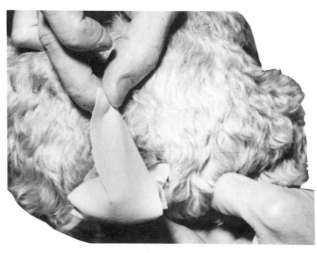

Figure 5–78 The opposite tape ends are similarly overlapped on the dorsal and lateral surfaces of the tail.

Figure 5–79 The second tape is applied at a 90° angle to the first and is overlapped on the lateral and ventral surfaces of the tail.

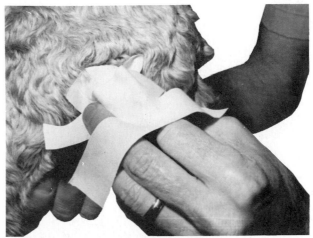

Figure 5–80 The opposite ends are similarly applied to overlap previous layers on the lateral and dorsal surfaces of the tail.

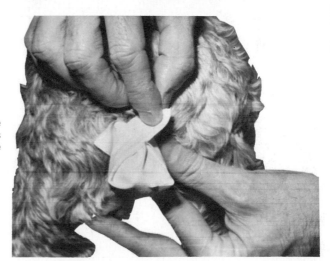

Figure 5–81 The tape ends are covered with a single circumferential tape; the result is a bandage that functions in much the same fashion as the Chinese finger basket puzzle.

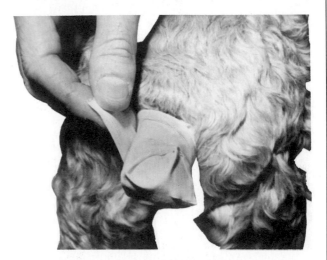

RESTRAINT DEVICES
The Sidebrace

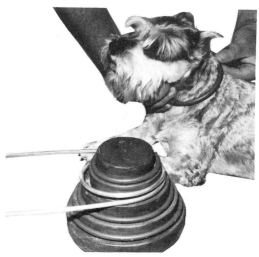

Figure 5–82 An aluminum rod is bent to an appropriately sized ring for the animal's neck by means of a wooden block and rubber sizing rings.

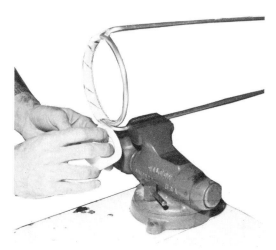

Figure 5–83 The ring is covered with adhesive tape applied with the adhesive side exposed.

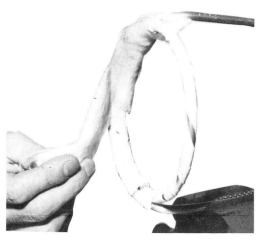

Figure 5–84 The reversed adhesive tape is covered with absorbent cotton.

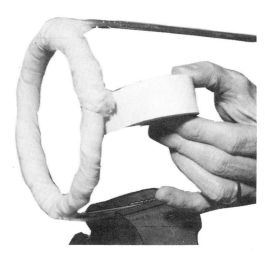

Figure 5–85 The absorbent cotton is covered with adhesive tape for even padding.

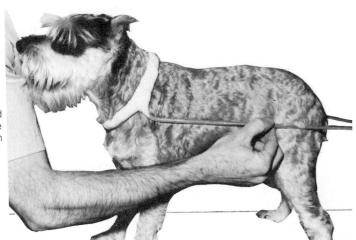

Figure 5–86 The aluminum rod is extended along the lateral surface of the shoulder, thorax, and abdomen to the flank.

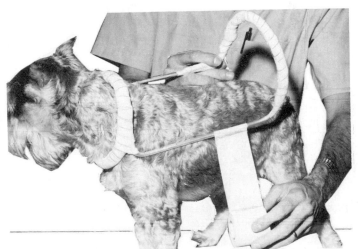

Figure 5–87 The aluminum rod is joined in a padded arch dorsal to the flank.

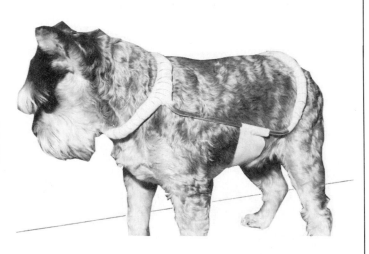

Figure 5–88 Adhesive tape is applied from the aluminum rod on one side and is passed across the abdomen to the aluminum rod on the opposite side for stability.

Elizabethan Collar

Plastic Elizabethan collars are commercially available for dogs and cats. In some forms the collar fits directly about the neck and is firmly fixed. One model provides straps for gauze placement around the neck.

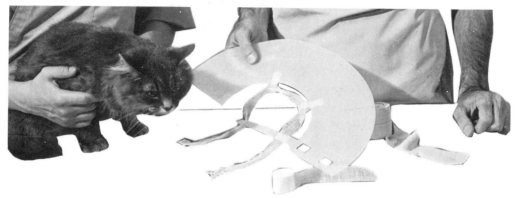

Figure 5–89   The plastic straps are formed, and gauze is threaded through the loops.

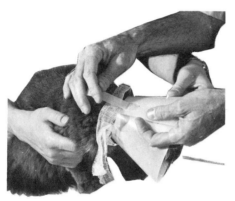

Figure 5–90   The collar is applied to fit snugly and is fixed in place with the appropriate strap.

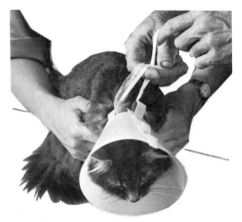

Figure 5–91 The gauze is tied around the neck.

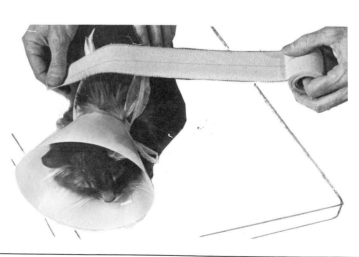

Figure 5–92 Strips of gauze are placed from the loops caudally and are fixed to the thorax with elastic adhesive tape.

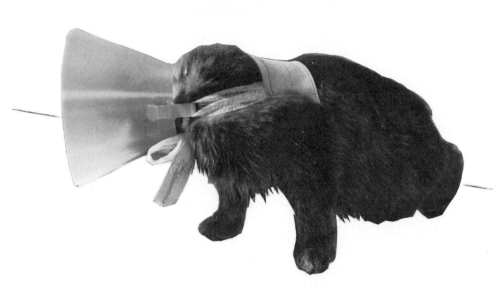

Figure 5–93 The collar should be large enough to cover the head. Fixation to a thoracic tape or halter is advised.

Foam Rubber Collar

Similar restraint from self-mutilation may be achieved with foam rubber. The ⅝ to ¾ inch foam is cut to fit the extended neck and is rolled around it.

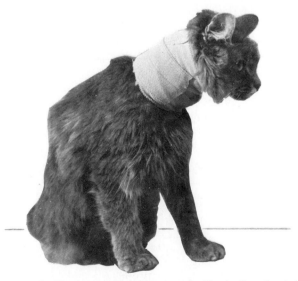

Figure 5–94 The foam rubber is wrapped with elastic adhesive tape.

REFERENCES

Brinker, W. O. and Sales, E. K.: Treatment of dislocation of the elbow in dogs. Vet. Med., 1949, *44*:135.

Cameron, D. B.: A simplified taping procedure to achieve upright ear carriage in dogs. Norden News, Winter/Spring, 1979, 26–27.

Cofield, R. B.: Technique in handling simple and compound fractures. North Am. Vet., 1934, *15*:32.

Ehmer, E. A.: Traumatic injuries in small animals. J.A.V.M.A., 1948, *112*:246.

Hickman, J.: *Veterinary Orthopaedics.* Edinburgh: Oliver and Boyd, 1964.

Knecht, C. D.: Application of temporary splints. Vet. Clin. North Am., 1975, 5(2):165–175.

Leonard, E. P.: *Fundamentals of Small Animal Surgery.* Philadelphia: W. B. Saunders Co., 1968.

Leonard, E. P.: *Orthopedic Surgery of the Dog and Cat,* 2nd ed. Philadelphia: W. B. Saunders Co., 1971.

Mason, C. T.: A new appliance for metacarpal and metatarsal surgery. Auburn Vet., 1948, *4*:91.

Olsen, M. L.: *Canine Surgery,* 4th ed. Evanston, Ill.: American Veterinary Publications, Inc., 1959.

Pozzi, L.: Treatment of fractures of the mandible in the dog. Atti. Soc. Ital. Sci. Vet., 1969, *14*:214.

Robinson, G. W., McCoy, L., and Gili, K. M.: Feline bandaging and splinting. Friskies Research Digest, 1978, *14*(3):4–5, 15.

Wagner, M., Lutsky, I., Becker, B., and Rodgers, R.: Clinical and research applications of a new elastic cohesive bandage. Am. J. Surg., 1970, *119*:298–299. The Yorke Medical Group.

Waterman, N. G., Stockinger, T., and Goldblatt, D.: Effects of various dressings on skin and subcutaneous temperatures. Arch. Surg., 1967, *95*:464.

6

WOUND DRESSING FOR THE HORSE

6

WOUND DRESSING FOR THE HORSE

EQUINE BANDAGING

Bandages are used for many purposes and are constructed of many types of materials. The choice of material will depend on the purpose of the bandage. Most bandages used on horses are applied to the lower extremities, although other areas can be bandaged.

Bandages are used to prevent trauma. There are several types: shipping bandages, standing bandages, run down bandages (to prevent trauma to the palmar area of the fetlocks), support bandages, sweat bandages, and medication bandages. The construction and application of the bandage is frequently tailored to the particular problem and to the individual case.

There are multiple choices of material, with cotton or some other bulk fiber used as padding. Rarely is a roll of bandage applied without padding. The padding helps to apply even pressure and helps to prevent slipping. The cotton may be used in a roll or in sheets. Thickness may vary with the amount used. The sheet or roll cotton may be used plain or may be covered with gauze. Quilted wraps constructed of washable cotton material are commercially available, as are wraps that have a foam rubber inner liner.

Many types of material are used to hold the leg wraps in place. Elastic gauze, tape and bandages, with or without ties on one end, and flannel are used. Flannel wraps are not commercially available. They can be made by tearing 5 in. to 6 in. strips of flannel from a bolt. Each strip should be approximately 11 ft. long. These flannel wraps are washable and can be used many times. The flannel wraps are secured in place with tape or large safety pins.

BANDAGING THE ABDOMEN AND TAIL
The Abdomen

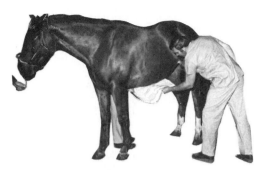

Figure 6–1 A sterile, nonadherent dressing is centered in an absorbent abdominal bandage and is placed under the ventral incision.

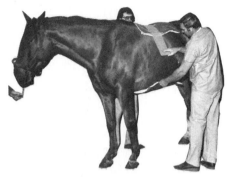

Figure 6–2 A similar dressing is placed on the back to prevent pressure sores.

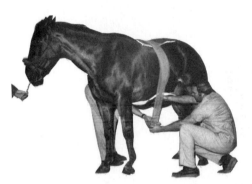

Figure 6–3 The bandages are covered with 3 to 4 inch wide roll gauze.

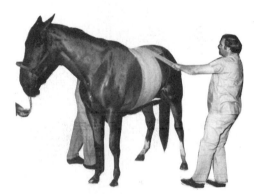

Figure 6–4 Roll gauze is applied tightly from cranial to caudal.

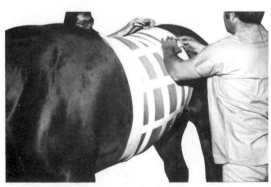

Figure 6–5 Two-inch tape is applied to prevent slippage. Elastic tape* is applied loosely to the hair and edges of the bandage.

*Elastikon Porous Adhesive Tape is manufactured by Johnson and Johnson, New Brunswick, N.J.

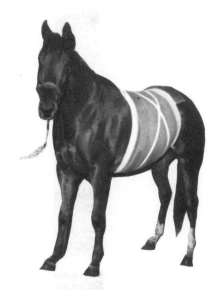

Figure 6–6 The tape may be crossed to prevent slippage.

The Tail Wrap

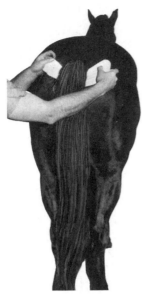

Figure   6–7 The   hair   is smoothed, and a 4 to 6 inch wide roll bandage is placed below the tail.

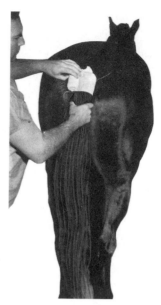

Figure 6–8 The wrap is locked by overlapping the first layer.

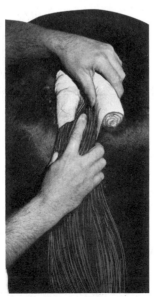

Figure 6–9 A small tuft of hair is pulled forward and is covered with the next overlapping layer to prevent slippage.

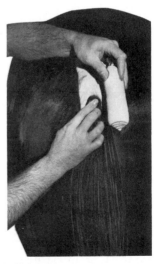

Figure 6–10 A tuft of hair is incorporated in the bandage every one to three wraps.

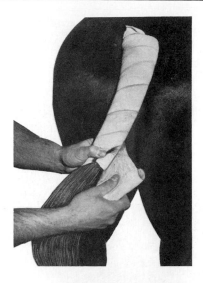

Figure 6–11 The tail is covered to the end of the vertebrae.

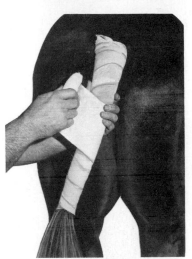

Figure 6–12 The bandage is continued by overlapping the wraps from the end cranially. The tail need not be wrapped so tightly as to impede the circulation because the hair is incorporated.

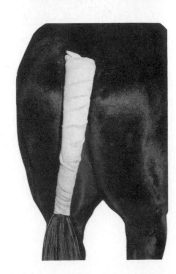

Figure 6–13 The end of the bandage is fixed with tape or a safety pin or is tucked between two layers.

BANDAGING THE HEAD AND NECK
The Head and Eye

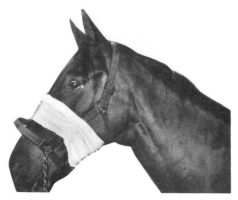

Figure 6–14 A section of large-diameter stockinette is rolled over the muzzle.

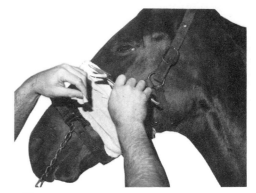

Figure 6–15 A hole is cut for the eye(s).

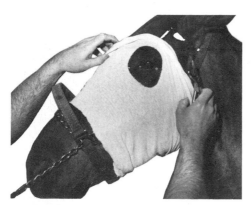

Figure 6–16 The stockinette is rolled over the eyes.

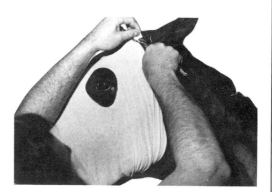

Figure 6–17 Holes are cut for the ears.

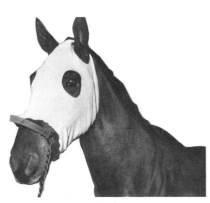

Figure 6–18 Elastic tape is applied loosely around the muzzle. Tape is not necessary at the top because of the ears. A halter is placed over the stockinette.

Neck Cradle

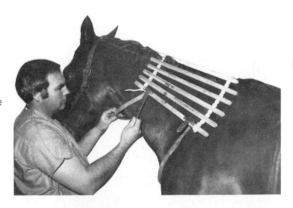

Figure 6–19 The cradle is placed over the neck, and the straps are fastened.

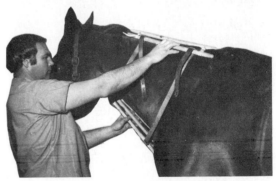

Figure 6–20 The cradle is rotated.

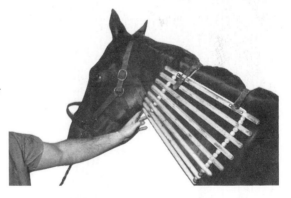

Figure 6–21 The straps are adjusted after the cradle is repositioned.

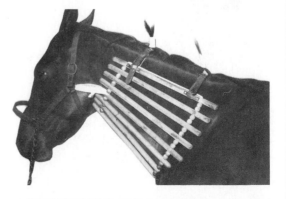

Figure 6–22 The cradle should be attached to the halter rings on each side. The mane is plaited or taped over the straps to prevent slippage.

BANDAGING THE EXTREMITIES
The Forelimb
The Foot

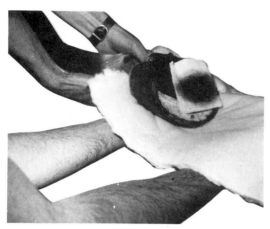

Figure 6–23 A length of Combine Roll° or roll cotton is applied over the medicated foot.

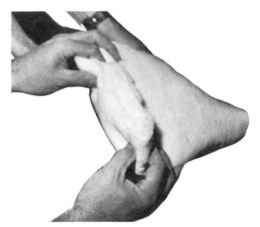

Figure 6–24 The padding is folded around the foot.

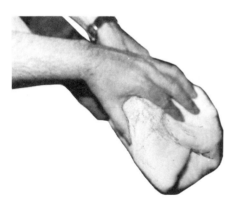

Figure 6–25 The edges of the roll are folded over the bottom of the foot.

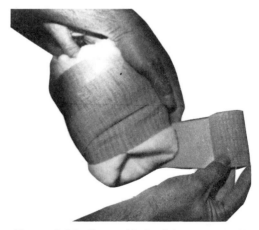

Figure 6–26 The padded roll is wrapped with elastic tape.

°Combine Roll is manufactured by Johnson and Johnson, New Brunswick, N.J.

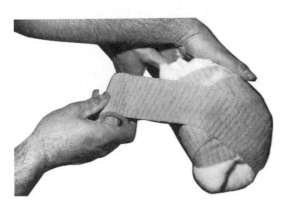

Figure 6–27 The elastic tape is rolled over the bulbs of the heel.

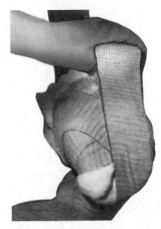

Figure 6–28 The elastic tape is continued to cover the toe.

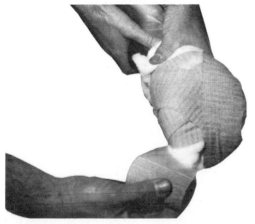

Figure 6–29 Taping continues around the heel and toe.

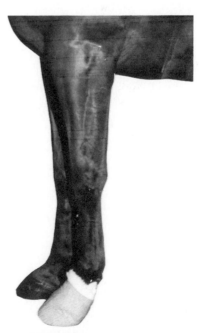

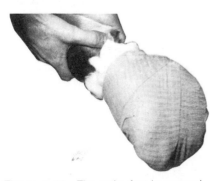

Figure 6–30 The entire foot is covered.

Figure 6–31 The elastic tape does not contact the coronary band, which is padded.

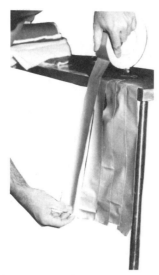

Figure 6–32 Strips of duct tape are stuck together to form a sheet.

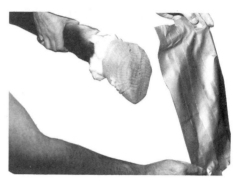

Figure 6–33 The sheet is prepared for application to the foot.

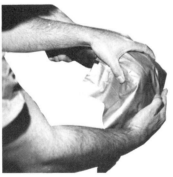

Figure 6–34 The duct tape is stuck to the bottom of the foot.

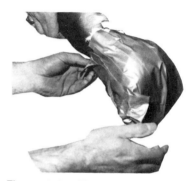

Figure 6–35 The duct tape is extended and is attached to the padded coronary band.

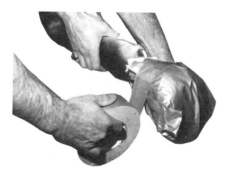

Figure 6–36 The entire foot is wrapped with a roll of duct tape to hold the bandage in place and to keep the foot dry.

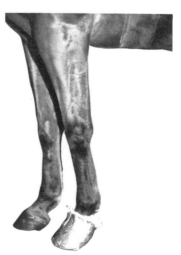

Figure 6–37 Excessive bandage may be trimmed.

Lower Leg Bandage — Construction

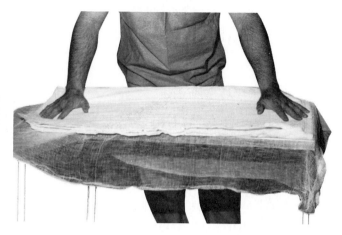

Figure 6–38 A leg bandage can be constructed by placing roll or sheet cotton in the middle of a larger piece of cheese-cloth.

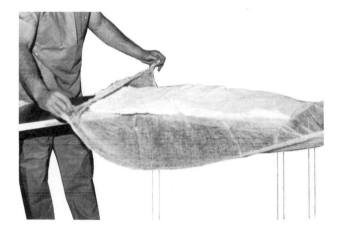

Figure 6–39 The ends are covered with cheesecloth.

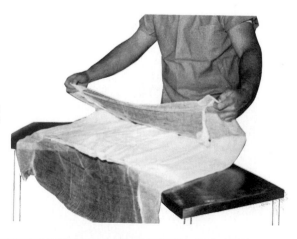

Figure 6–40 The sides of the cheesecloth are folded over the cotton. The finished bandage is rolled for use or wrapped and autoclaved.

Lower Leg Bandage — Application

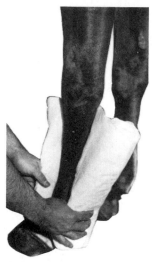

Figure 6–41 The bandage is wrapped clockwise on the left leg or counterclockwise on the right.

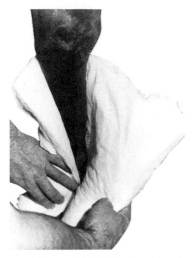

Figure 6–42 The bandage is carefully overlapped from the bottom proximally to provide a smooth surface.

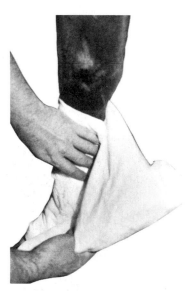

Figure 6–43 The top of the bandage is tucked in.

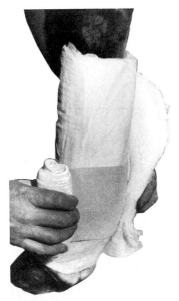

Figure 6–44 The end of a flannel roll bandage, 4 inches or more wide, is inserted between the layers of the fabricated leg bandage.

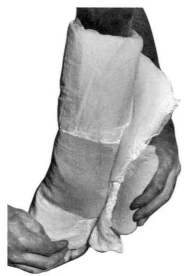

Figure 6–45 The flannel roll is wrapped to overlap the end.

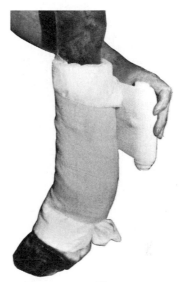

Figure 6–46 The flannel roll is wrapped to the top of the bandage and is returned distally.

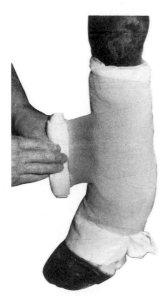

Figure 6–47 The flannel wrap should end at the midshaft.

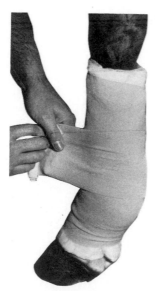

Figure 6–48 The flannel bandage should end or should be folded to end on the lateral side.

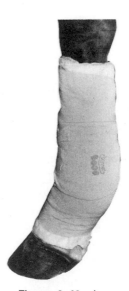

Figure 6–49 A complete lower leg bandage.

Knee Bandage — Construction

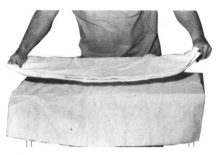

Figure 6–50 A knee bandage can be fabricated from roll or sheet cotton and cheesecloth. The first sheet of cotton is unfolded. Two or three full-thickness cotton sheets are centered on the unfolded piece.

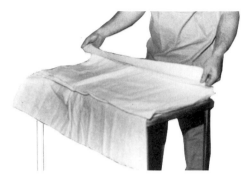

Figure 6–51 One edge of the unfolded cotton sheet is folded over the full-thickness sheets.

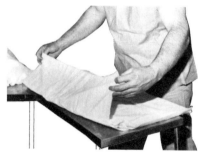

Figure 6–52 The other edge is folded, and all wrinkles are removed.

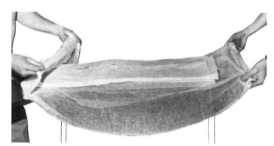

Figure 6–53 The cotton composite is centered on a larger piece of cheesecloth, and the ends are folded.

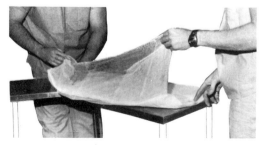

Figure 6–54 The sides of the cheesecloth are folded, and the bandage is smoothed.

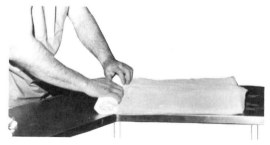

Figure 6–55 The bandage is rolled and is ready for use or sterilization by autoclaving.

Spider Bandage — Construction

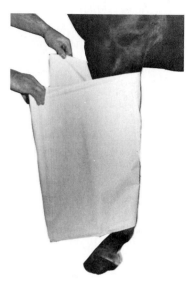

Figure 6–56 The spider bandage, also called a many tie or many tail bandage, is fabricated from a sheet of muslin or flannel measured to cover the leg and padding. Spider bandages may be washed and reused.

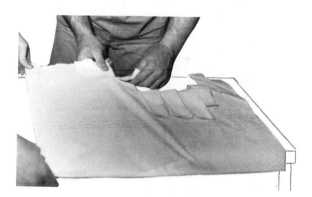

Figure 6–57 The sheet is cut to the desired length and is folded lengthwise. Cuts are made 1½ inches apart on the doubled side with bandage scissors. The cloth is carefully torn to form tie ends.

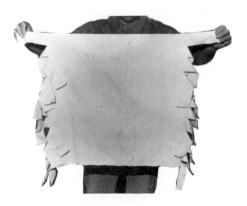

Figure 6–58 The finished spider bandage.

Knee Bandage — Application

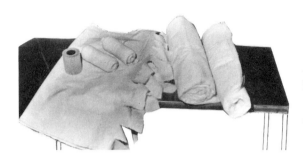

Figure 6–59 The materials needed for a forelimb bandage that extends above the knee include one rolled low leg bandage, one longer knee bandage, a spider bandage, two rolls of stretch track bandage or gauze, and elastic tape.

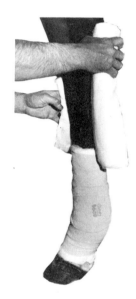

Figure 6-60 A lower leg bandage is applied (Figs. 6–41 to 6–49). The knee bandage is positioned to overlap the lower leg bandage by 2 inches and to extend at least 6 inches above the knee. The size can be varied during construction to fit the limb.

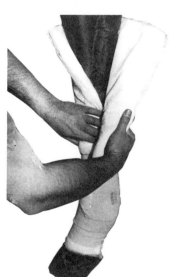

Figure 6–61 Beginning distally, the bandage is overlapped and is wrapped around the leg as tightly as possible.

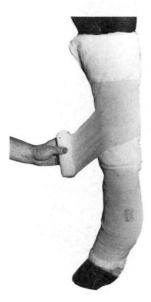

Figure 6–62 The elastic bandage is tucked under the middle of the overlapped bandage and is fully wrapped. All wrinkles are removed before continuing application. The elastic bandage is applied snugly but not tight enough to prevent flexion of the knee.

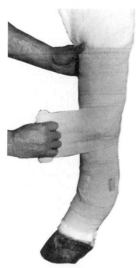

Figure 6–63 The elastic roll is applied proximally to above the knee and distally to the lower leg bandage. A firm grip and even pressure are maintained to prevent wrinkling.

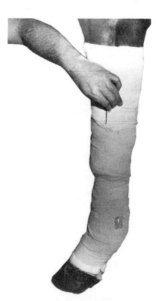

Figure 6–64 The elastic wrap is continued to the proximal end and is returned to the starting point. The end is secured with pins or tape.

Spider Bandage — Application

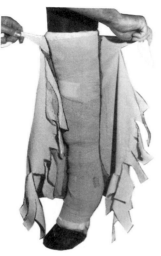

Figure 6–65 The spider bandage is applied over a knee bandage, maintaining position but allowing knee motion.

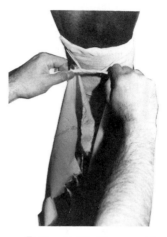

Figure 6–66 The spider bandage is placed on the medial side of the leg, and the top strands are tied. A bow is tied over a half-hitch.

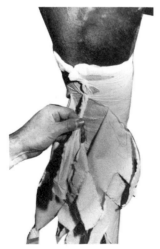

Figure 6–67 The ends are twisted to prevent loosening.

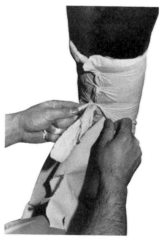

Figure 6–68 The next lower half-hitch is placed over the twisted ties.

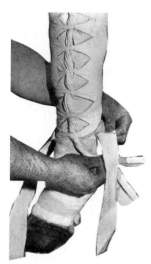

Figure 6–69 The long ends are tucked proximally before the last tie.

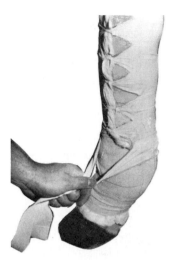

Figure 6–70 The distal tie is tightened.

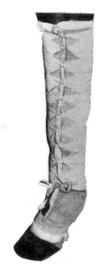

Figure 6–71 A bow is applied over the tightened half-hitch.

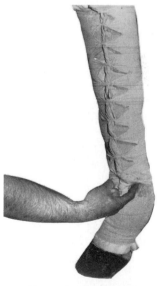

Figure 6–72 The ends and loops are tucked under the edge of the bandage and are covered with a section of adhesive tape. The entire bandage can be removed in reverse order and reapplied if it is not soiled.

The Rearlimb
Lower Leg Bandage — Application

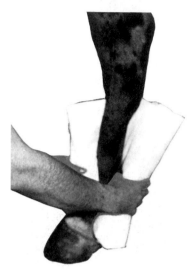

Figure 6–73 Fabrication of the lower leg bandage is illustrated in Figures 6–38 to 6–40. The bandage is applied smoothly around the leg with even pressure.

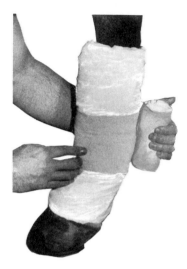

Figure 6–74 A roll of elastic gauze or track wrap is locked in the middle of the overlapping bandage.

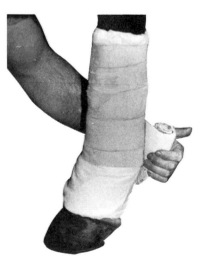

Figure 6–75 The elastic roll is wrapped proximally to the top and then distally to the bottom of the bandage.

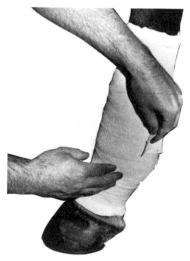

Figure 6–76 The elastic wrap should end in the middle of the bandage on the lateral side. The end is secured with pins or tape.

Hock Bandage — Application

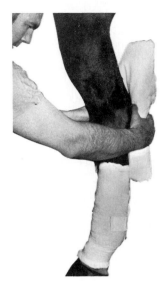
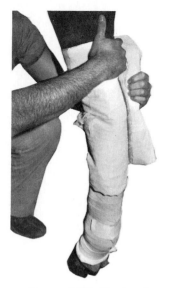
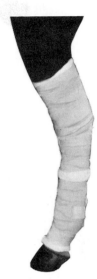

Figure 6–77 The hock bandage is applied over the lower leg bandage.

Figure 6–78 The bandage is smoothed and tucked under the outer wrap.

Figure 6–79 Elastic gauze or wrap is used to cover the bandage.

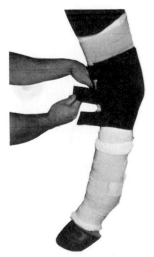
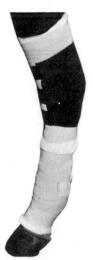

Figure 6–80 A commercial hock bandage with Velcro closure can be used to hold the bandage in place.

Figure 6–81 A hock bandage with Velcro closure.

Spider Bandage — Application

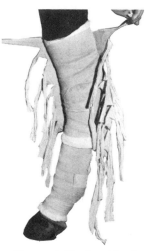

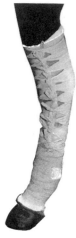

Figure 6–82 A spider bandage may be applied to prevent slippage.

Figure 6–83 The spider bandage is applied with the ties on the lateral or caudal aspect of the limb.

Robert Jones Bandage

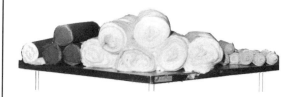

Figure 6–84 The materials needed for a Robert Jones bandage for an adult horse include 10 one pound rolls of absorbent cotton, six elastic wraps, and tape.

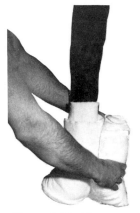

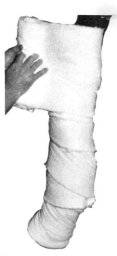

Figure 6-85 The cotton is rolled on the leg from the foot proximally. Removal of the paper lining facilitates application.

Figure 6–86 The leg is wrapped by overlapping the absorbent cotton.

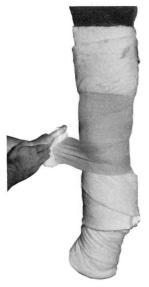

Figure 6–87 Elastic wrap is applied to hold the cotton in place.

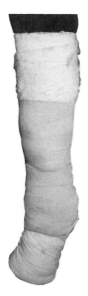

Figure 6–88 The wrap is overlapped snugly from bottom to top.

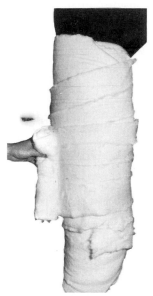

Figure 6–89 Additional alternate layers of cotton and elastic wrap are applied until the full 10 pounds of cotton are applied.

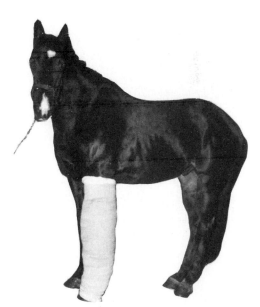

Figure 6–90 A completed Robert Jones bandage.

7

APPLICATION OF TECHNIQUES

7

APPLICATION OF TECHNIQUES

INTRODUCTION

It is not the intent of this text to present specific surgical techniques. The following procedures are presented to demonstrate the use of instruments, sutures, suture patterns, and fundamental techniques that are common to many surgical procedures. In each instance, the operative procedure is neither exclusive nor unique. In each instance, it is simply one means of performing the surgery that has proved satisfactory and that may best present the proper use of good fundamental surgical techniques.

In each operative procedure the animal has been sedated and anesthesia has been induced with a short-acting intravenous barbiturate or with inhalant anesthetic and a face mask. The animal is subsequently intubated, and anesthesia is maintained with an inhalant anesthetic in combination with oxygen.

OVARIOHYSTERECTOMY

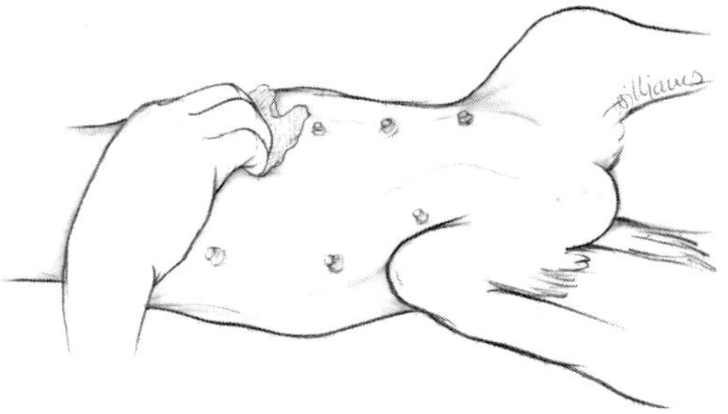

Figure 7–1 The animal is placed in dorsal recumbency. A broad surgical area is clipped and prepared for aseptic surgery with a repeated surgical scrub. The scrub agent should be povidone-iodine.

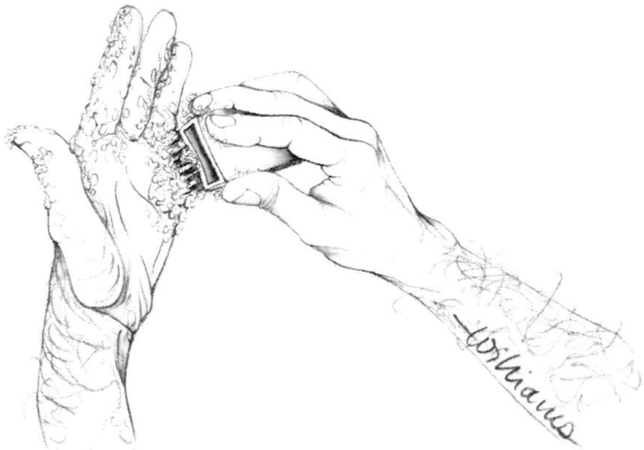

Figure 7–2 As the animal is prepared for aseptic surgery, the surgeon prepares himself by completely cleaning the fingernails and by performing no less than two thorough surgical scrubs and rinses. Each surface of each finger of each hand is thoroughly scrubbed for a total of no less than five minutes.

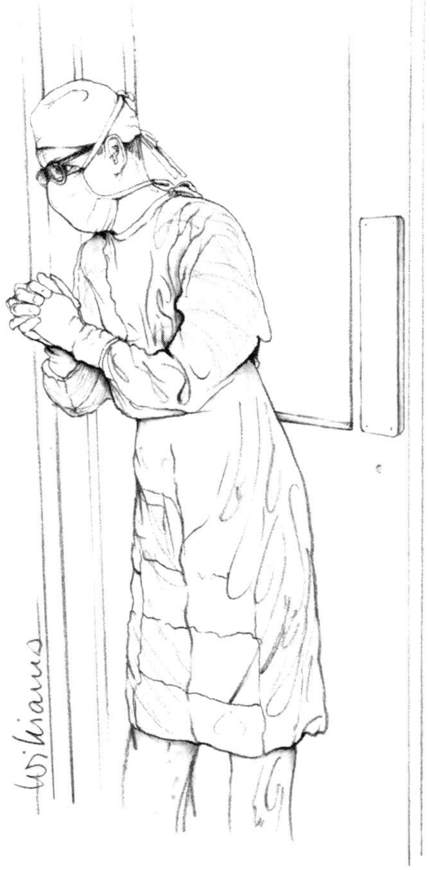

Figure 7-3 The gowned and gloved surgeon joins the patient in the operative suite for the surgical procedure.

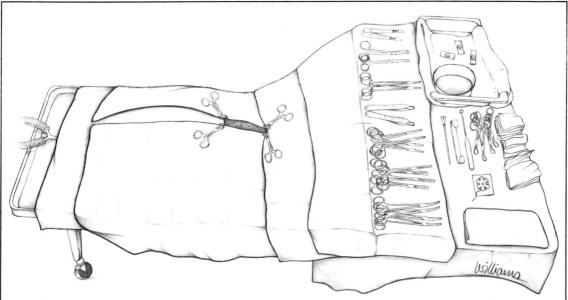

Figure 7–4 Disposable drapes are used to cover the instrument stand, patient, and operating table. The drapes are placed so that no pocket is present for possible contamination during the operative procedure.

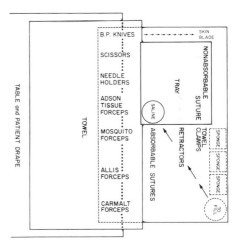

Figure 7–5 A scheme for the organization of surgical instruments on the instrument table is presented. Such a uniform arrangement of instruments provides each surgeon in the operating room with an awareness of the presence and availability of instruments found in standard packs. The simple organization of instruments in a uniform and consistent pattern saves time and effort for the operating surgeon.

Figure 7–6 A #10 Bard-Parker scalpel is used to incise the skin in the first step of the operative procedure.

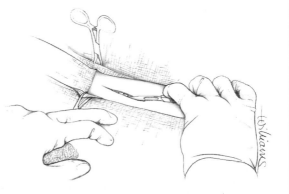

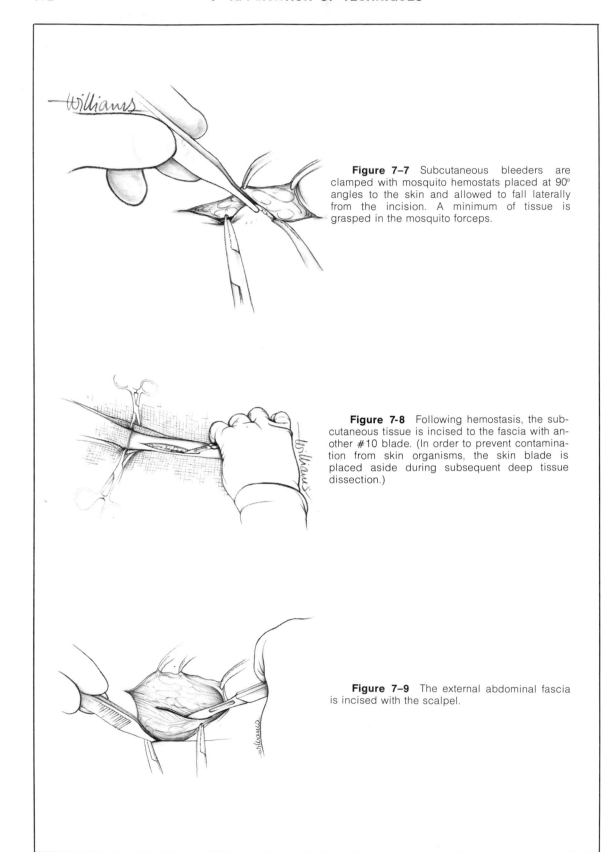

Figure 7–7 Subcutaneous bleeders are clamped with mosquito hemostats placed at 90° angles to the skin and allowed to fall laterally from the incision. A minimum of tissue is grasped in the mosquito forceps.

Figure 7-8 Following hemostasis, the subcutaneous tissue is incised to the fascia with another #10 blade. (In order to prevent contamination from skin organisms, the skin blade is placed aside during subsequent deep tissue dissection.)

Figure 7–9 The external abdominal fascia is incised with the scalpel.

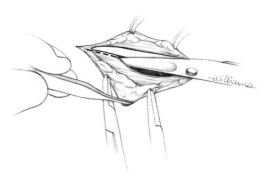

Figure 7–10 The fascial incision is extended cranially and caudally with scissors.

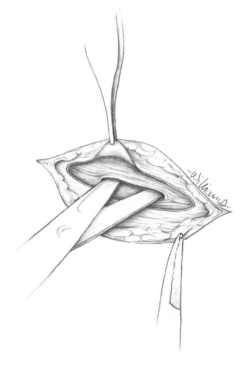

Figure 7–11 The abdominal muscle is separated by blunt dissection. This is performed by introducing the scissors through the muscle fibers and opening the scissor blades.

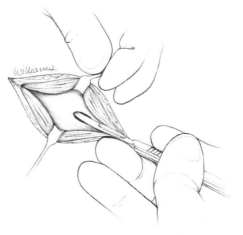

Figure 7–12 The peritoneum is exposed as the abdominal muscles are retracted with Senn retractors. The surgeon makes a small incision in the peritoneum with a lifting motion of the deep scalpel.

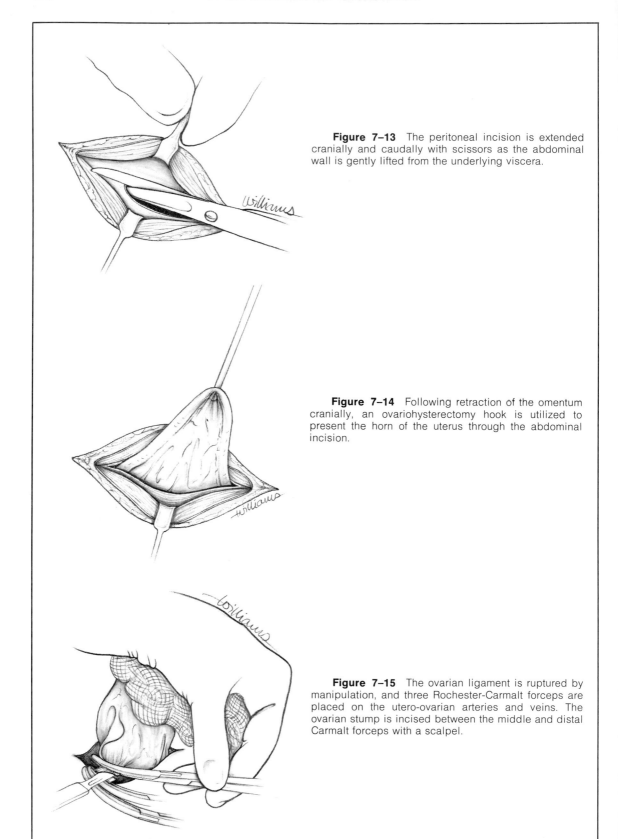

Figure 7–13 The peritoneal incision is extended cranially and caudally with scissors as the abdominal wall is gently lifted from the underlying viscera.

Figure 7–14 Following retraction of the omentum cranially, an ovariohysterectomy hook is utilized to present the horn of the uterus through the abdominal incision.

Figure 7–15 The ovarian ligament is ruptured by manipulation, and three Rochester-Carmalt forceps are placed on the utero-ovarian arteries and veins. The ovarian stump is incised between the middle and distal Carmalt forceps with a scalpel.

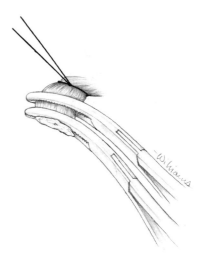

Figure 7–16 A single 2–0 medium chromic catgut ligature is placed no less than 4 mm from the proximal Carmalt forceps. The gut is tied and the ends are cut.

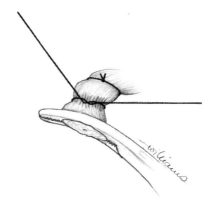

Figure 7–17 A second 2–0 medium catgut ligature is placed at the point where the proximal Carmalt forceps have crushed the ovarian stump.

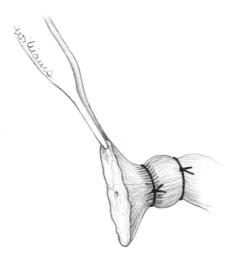

Figure 7–18 The stump is checked for bleeding. Each pedicle should be checked and returned to the abdominal cavity.

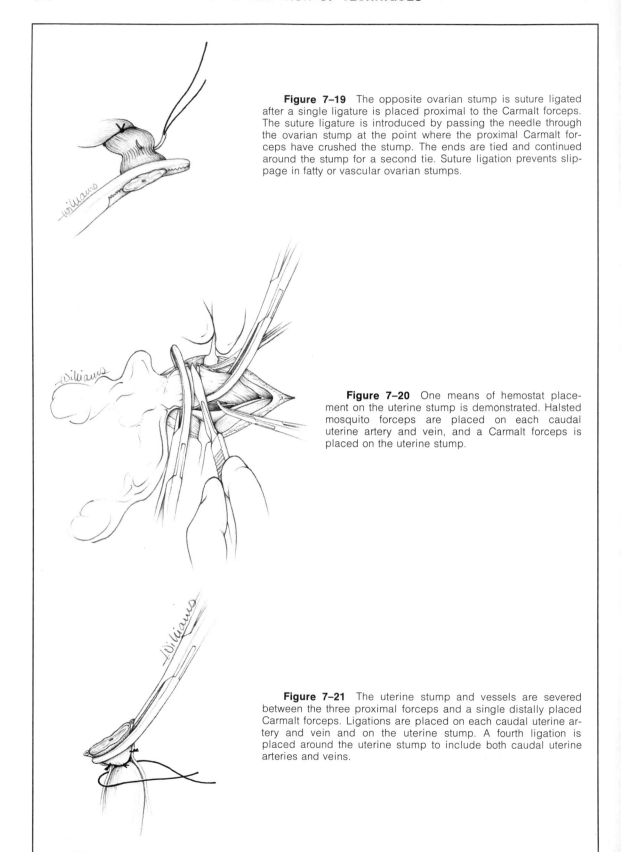

Figure 7–19 The opposite ovarian stump is suture ligated after a single ligature is placed proximal to the Carmalt forceps. The suture ligature is introduced by passing the needle through the ovarian stump at the point where the proximal Carmalt forceps have crushed the stump. The ends are tied and continued around the stump for a second tie. Suture ligation prevents slippage in fatty or vascular ovarian stumps.

Figure 7–20 One means of hemostat placement on the uterine stump is demonstrated. Halsted mosquito forceps are placed on each caudal uterine artery and vein, and a Carmalt forceps is placed on the uterine stump.

Figure 7–21 The uterine stump and vessels are severed between the three proximal forceps and a single distally placed Carmalt forceps. Ligations are placed on each caudal uterine artery and vein and on the uterine stump. A fourth ligation is placed around the uterine stump to include both caudal uterine arteries and veins.

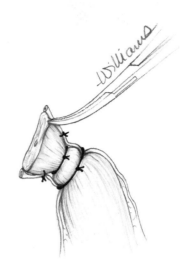

Figure 7–22 The hemostats are removed, and the stump is checked for bleeding.

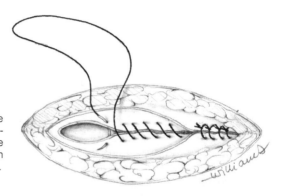

Figure 7–23 Following replacement of the uterine stump in the abdomen, the peritoneum is apposed with 2–0 medium chromic catgut in a simple continuous pattern, and the fascia is sutured with similar suture material in a simple interrupted pattern.

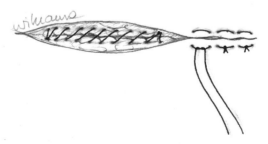

Figure 7–24 The subcutaneous tissue is closed with a simple continuous or running suture of 2–0 or 3–0 medium chromic catgut. The skin is apposed with a nonabsorbable suture material in a horizontal mattress pattern.

UMBILICAL HERNIORRHAPHY

The species of the patient alters the size and arrangement of the surgical suite. The principles of asepsis and good surgical techniques do not vary.

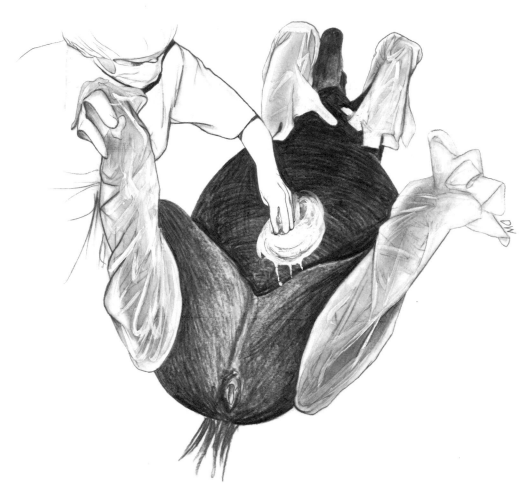

Figure 7–25 The horse is placed in dorsal recumbency, and the limbs are covered with disposable rectal examination gloves. The clipped abdomen is scrubbed three times from the hernia outward with povidone-iodine surgical scrub and is rinsed between each scrub. A final povidone-iodine spray is applied.

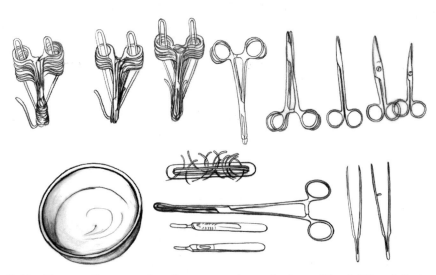

Figure 7–26 After aseptic preparation, the surgeon drapes the horse (Fig. 1–54) and displays the surgical instruments on a table covered with double sterile drapes. A standard table setup is used.

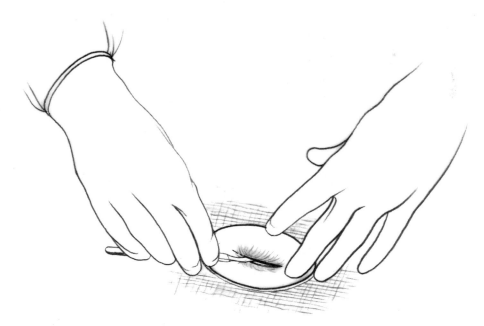

Figure 7–27 A longitudinal skin incision is made over the hernia with a #21 blade on a #4 Bard-Parker handle.

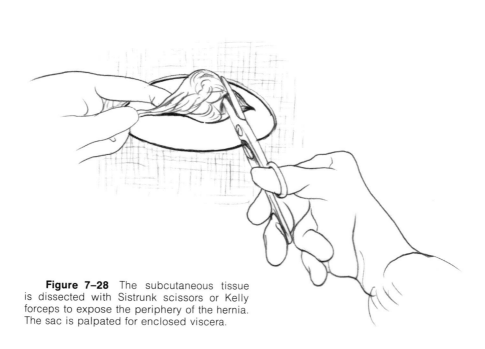

Figure 7–28 The subcutaneous tissue is dissected with Sistrunk scissors or Kelly forceps to expose the periphery of the hernia. The sac is palpated for enclosed viscera.

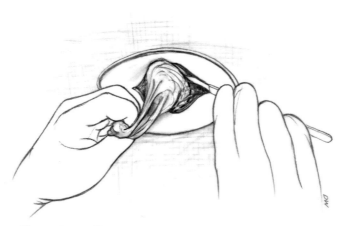

Figure 7–29 The circumference of the hernia is incised with a deep scalpel, and the redundant tissue is excised or replaced in the abdominal cavity.

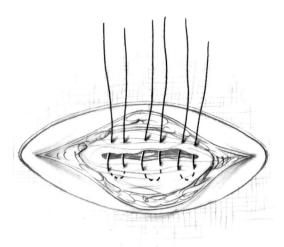

Figure 7–30 The abdominal incision is closed by the placement of Mayo mattress sutures with size 1 or 2 medium chromic catgut.

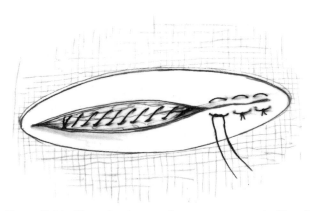

Figure 7–31 The subcutaneous tissues are apposed with a simple continuous suture of 0 catgut. The skin is sutured with nonabsorbable suture using a vertical mattress suture pattern.

REPAIR OF FRACTURED FEMUR BY INTRAMEDULLARY PINNING

Intramedullary fixation of a fractured femur by open surgical approach is demonstrated as an illustration of the use of instruments in orthopedic procedures. The technique is only one of the many techniques available for fracture repair and is not the only procedure that could be used in the type of fracture demonstrated.

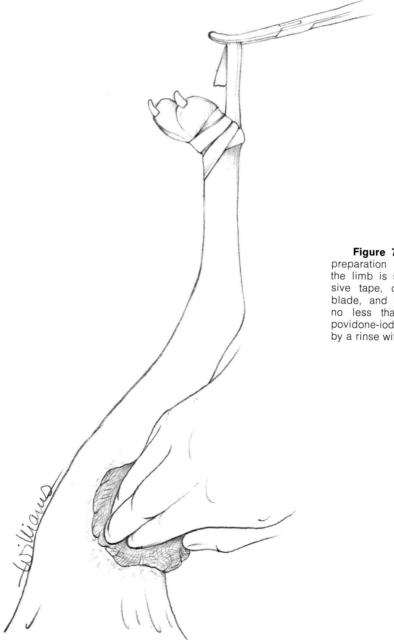

Figure 7–32 As part of the preparation for aseptic surgery, the limb is suspended by adhesive tape, clipped with a #40 blade, and thoroughly scrubbed no less than three times with povidone-iodine scrub followed by a rinse with alcohol.

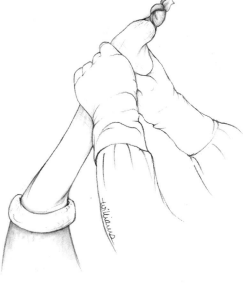

Figure 7–33 An assistant cuts the suspending adhesive tape and holds the limb while the surgeon applies a double-layered sterile stockinette to the foot. The stockinette is unrolled toward the thigh. In many instances, the non-sterile area of the foot is covered with a plastic sterile drape before application of the stockinette.

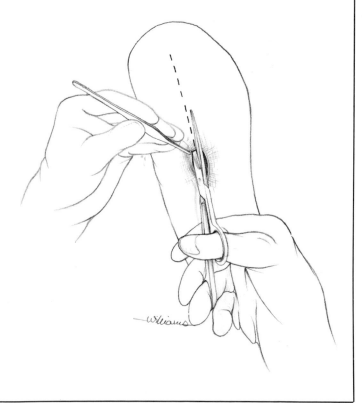

Figure 7–34 After complete draping of the animal, including apposition of the stockinette and disposable drapes in the region of the thigh, the stockinette is incised with scissors for the entire length of the proposed skin incision.

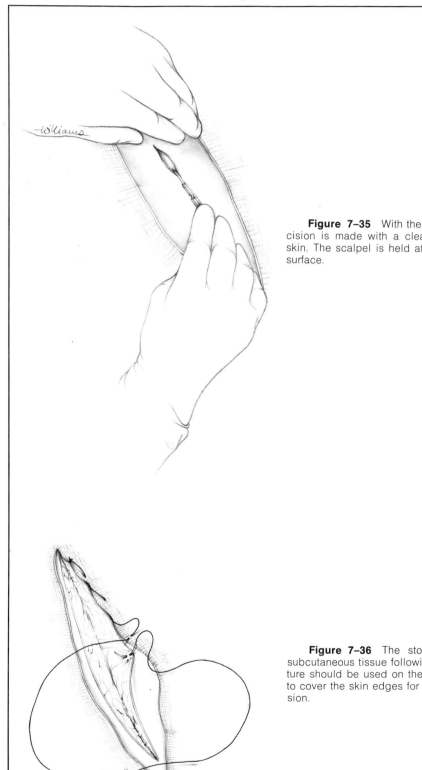

Figure 7–35 With the stockinette retracted, an incision is made with a clean, swift stroke through the skin. The scalpel is held at an acute angle to the skin surface.

Figure 7–36 The stockinette is sutured to the subcutaneous tissue following incision. An inverting suture should be used on the stockinette as it is applied to cover the skin edges for the entire length of the incision.

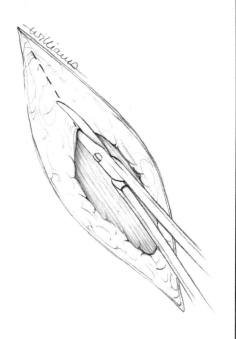

Figure 7–37 The subcutaneous tissue is incised with a scalpel or scissors to expose the underlying muscle fascia.

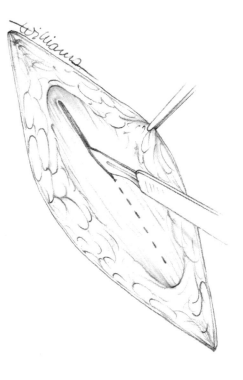

Figure 7–38 The fascia lata is incised with a scalpel in a continuous motion.

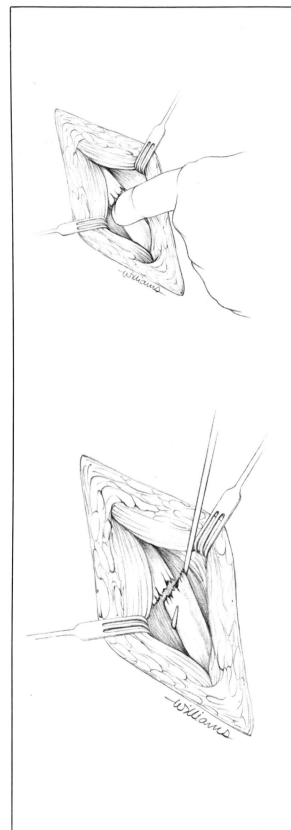

Figure 7–39 The muscles are separated by blunt dissection with Mayo or Metzenbaum scissors. Muscle retractors are placed in the incision, and the fracture site is exposed. Hematomas and fibrous tissue may be removed from the edges of the fractured fragments.

Figure 7–40 A bone hook is used to retract the ends of the fractured fragments for adequate visualization.

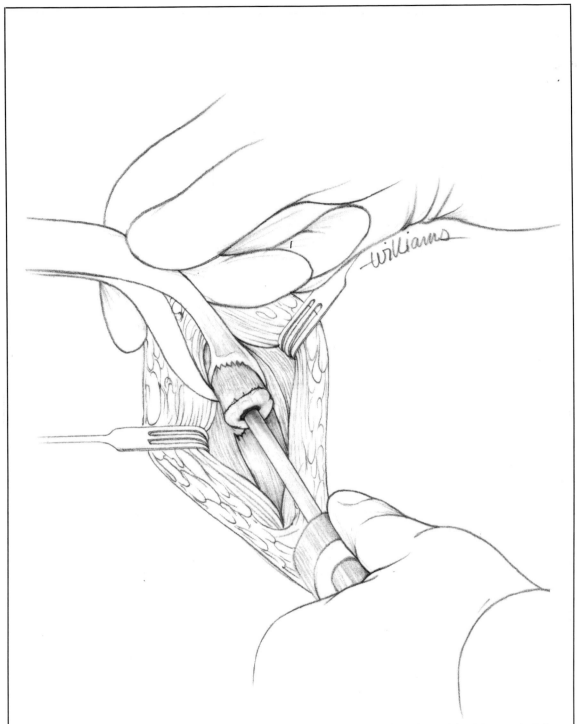

Figure 7–41 A Steinmann pin is placed by retrograde introduction into the proximal fragment of the femur. A Jacob's hand chuck is used to introduce the pin. The proximal bone end is held with Verbrugge bone holding forceps.

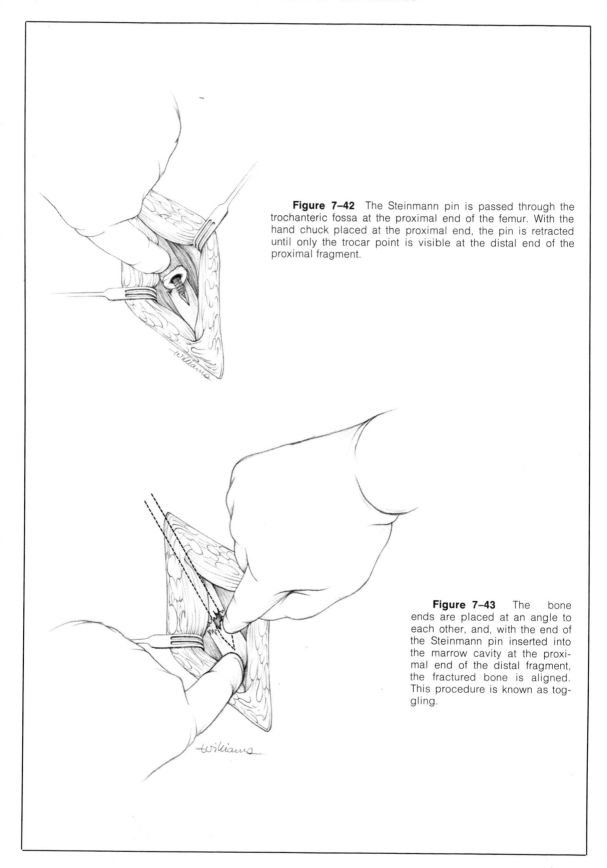

Figure 7–42 The Steinmann pin is passed through the trochanteric fossa at the proximal end of the femur. With the hand chuck placed at the proximal end, the pin is retracted until only the trocar point is visible at the distal end of the proximal fragment.

Figure 7–43 The bone ends are placed at an angle to each other, and, with the end of the Steinmann pin inserted into the marrow cavity at the proximal end of the distal fragment, the fractured bone is aligned. This procedure is known as toggling.

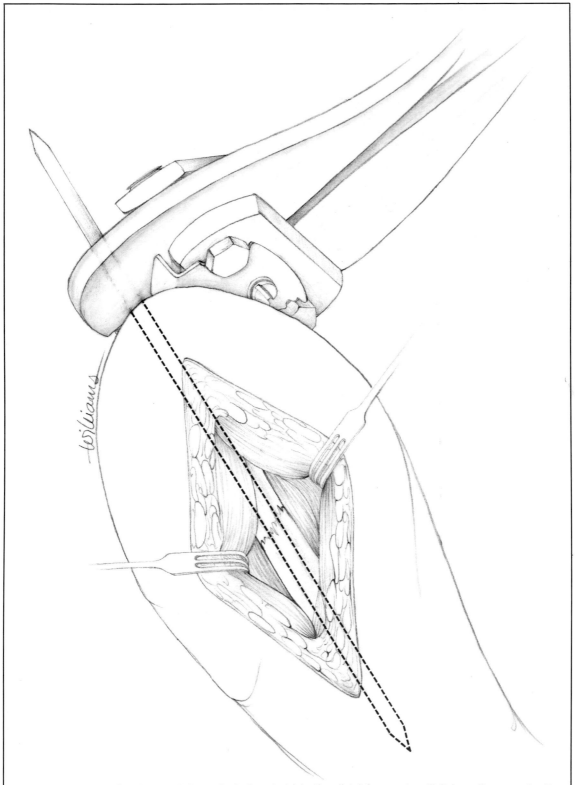

Figure 7–44 The intramedullary pin is inserted into the distal fragment until it is well apposed with cortical bone. The proximal exposed pin is cut at the skin surface with a pin cutter.

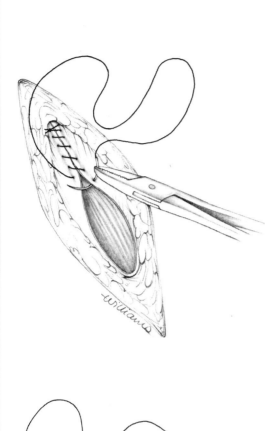

Figure 7–45 The muscle tissue is allowed to return around the bone. Periosteum that may have been loosened during the surgical approach is sutured with 2–0 or 3–0 catgut. The fascia lata is sutured with a simple continuous layer of 2–0 medium chromic catgut.

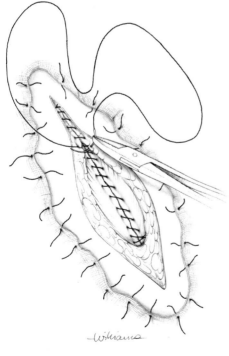

Figure 7–46 The stockinette sutures are cut, and the subcutaneous tissue is apposed with a simple continuous or simple running suture of 2–0 medium chromic catgut. The sutures should be placed so as to obliterate space and should be tacked to the underlying fascial layer.

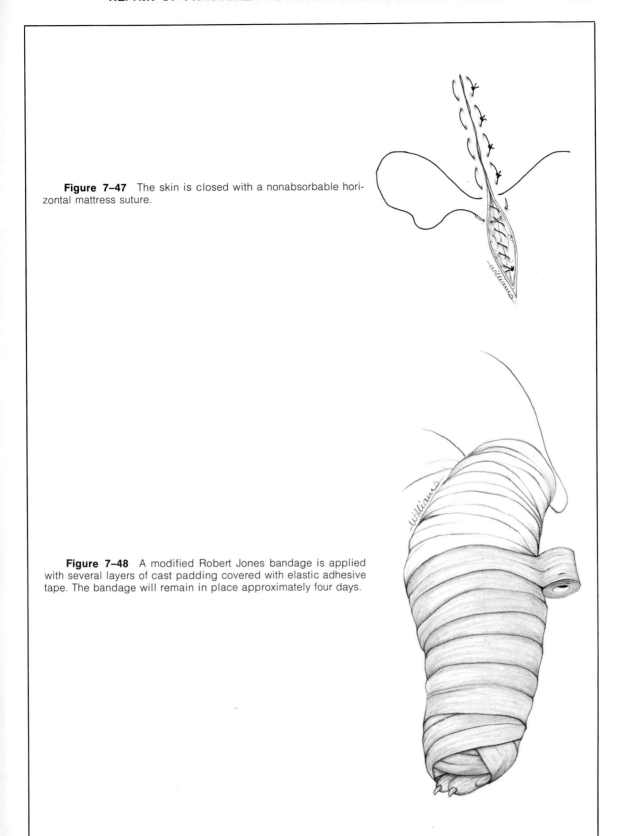

Figure 7–47 The skin is closed with a nonabsorbable horizontal mattress suture.

Figure 7–48 A modified Robert Jones bandage is applied with several layers of cast padding covered with elastic adhesive tape. The bandage will remain in place approximately four days.

REPAIR OF FRACTURED SMALL
METACARPAL BONE

Fracture of the small metacarpal bone results in a non-union with decreased function. The demonstrated repair includes excision of the distal fractured fragment and fixation of the proximal fragment with an orthopedic screw. The screw fixation is not needed if the fracture is more distal than the midpoint of the bone.

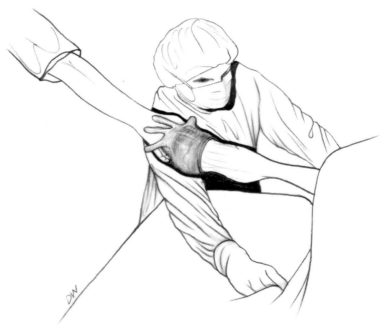

Figure 7–49 The lower leg is prepared for aseptic surgery with a disposable glove covering the cleaned hoof. The upper limb and body and the table below the leg are covered with sterile drapes.

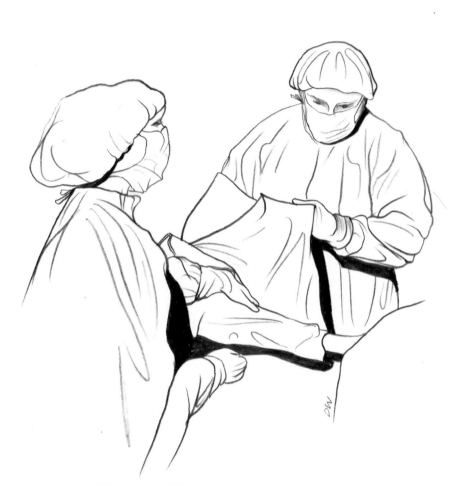

Figure 7–50   The foot is wrapped with a third drape.

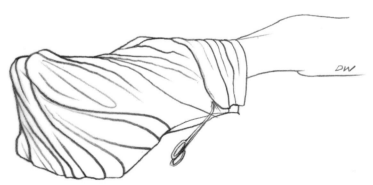

Figure 7–51   The foot drape is fixed with a Backhaus towel clamp.

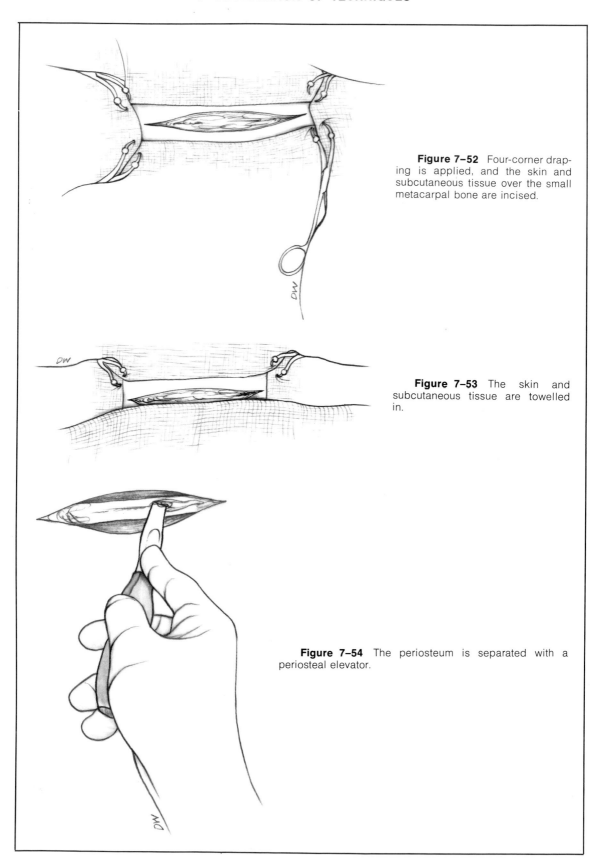

Figure 7–52 Four-corner draping is applied, and the skin and subcutaneous tissue over the small metacarpal bone are incised.

Figure 7–53 The skin and subcutaneous tissue are towelled in.

Figure 7–54 The periosteum is separated with a periosteal elevator.

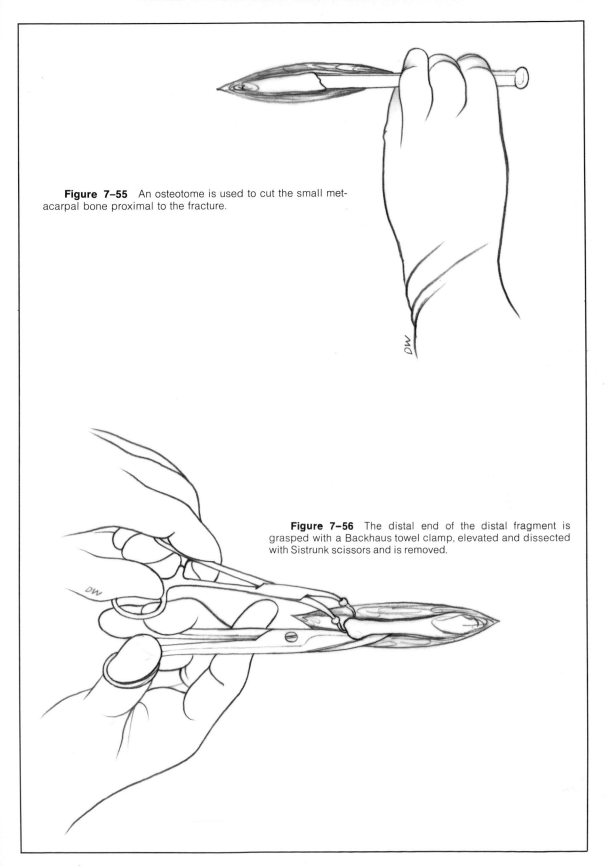

Figure 7–55 An osteotome is used to cut the small metacarpal bone proximal to the fracture.

Figure 7–56 The distal end of the distal fragment is grasped with a Backhaus towel clamp, elevated and dissected with Sistrunk scissors and is removed.

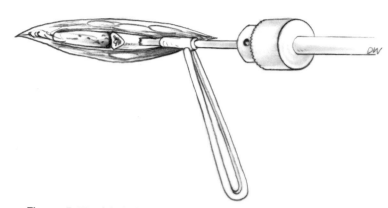

Figure 7–57   A hole is drilled in the remaining proximal fragment with a 4.5 mm drill bit through a 4.5 mm drill guide.

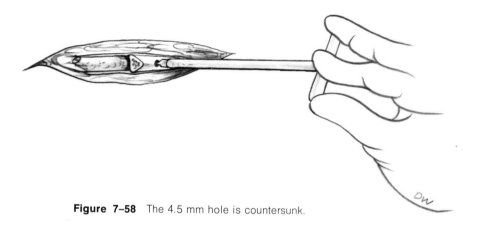

Figure 7–58   The 4.5 mm hole is countersunk.

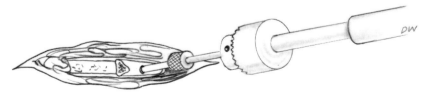

Figure 7–59   A 3.2 mm drill sleeve is placed in the 4.5 mm hole, and one cortex of the large metacarpal bone is drilled with a 3.2 mm drill bit.

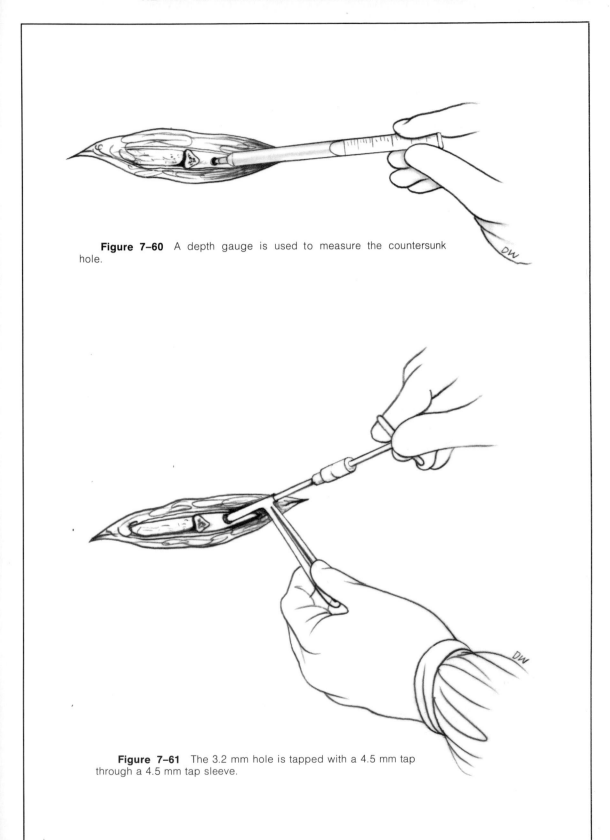

Figure 7–60 A depth gauge is used to measure the countersunk hole.

Figure 7–61 The 3.2 mm hole is tapped with a 4.5 mm tap through a 4.5 mm tap sleeve.

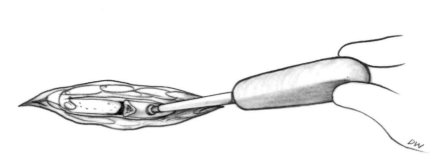

Figure 7–62 The appropriate length 4.5 mm cortical screw is applied finger-tight.

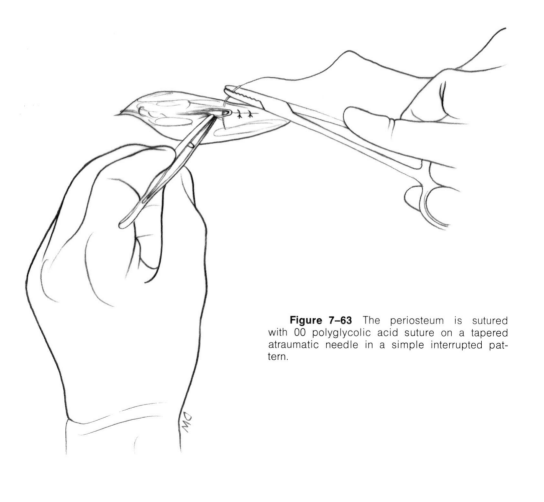

Figure 7–63 The periosteum is sutured with 00 polyglycolic acid suture on a tapered atraumatic needle in a simple interrupted pattern.

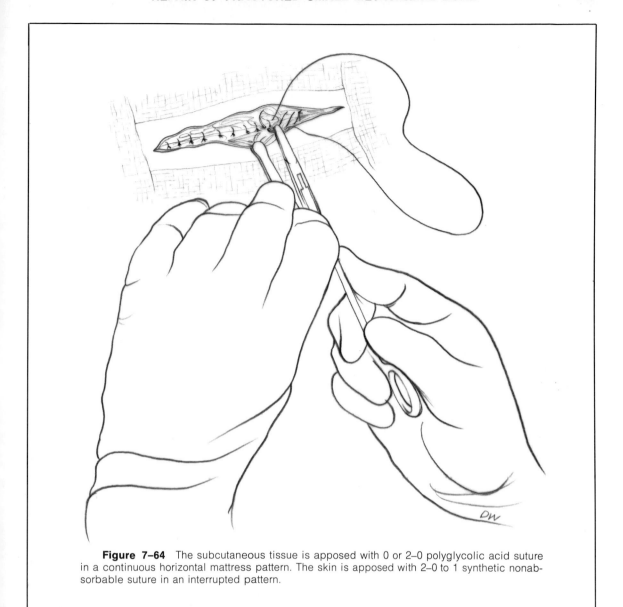

Figure 7–64   The subcutaneous tissue is apposed with 0 or 2–0 polyglycolic acid suture in a continuous horizontal mattress pattern. The skin is apposed with 2–0 to 1 synthetic nonabsorbable suture in an interrupted pattern.

SUMMARY

Each of the procedures demonstrated must be performed with adequate aseptic technique, correct use of instruments, and proper procedures. With aseptic technique and minimal trauma, optimum healing should result.

8

CASTS AND
SPLINTS FOR
SMALL ANIMALS

8

CASTS AND SPLINTS FOR SMALL ANIMALS

Many limb fractures of small animals may be successfully treated by simple reduction and immobilization. Proper immobilization may be achieved by external fixation in the form of coaptation splints, plaster of Paris casts, or the modified Thomas splint. Many factors must be considered in the determination of the means of fracture fixation. The location and type of fracture, the age and temperament of the animal, and the likelihood of confinement by the owner are a few of the factors to be considered. No single factor is sufficient to establish a specific treatment.

External fixation has certain advantages over internal fixation: (1) the original hematoma is maintained; (2) there is less risk of infection; (3) tissue trauma caused by a surgical approach is avoided; and (4) the procedure is less costly. There are, of course, disadvantages to external fixation as well: (1) reduction is less precise; (2) exercise and use of the limb muscles is limited; (3) disuse atrophy is more likely; and (4) aftercare is often more difficult.

A complete discussion of the indications for the use of splints is beyond the scope of this text. The guidelines presented here are general; the reader is referred to other texts on surgery for specific applications in the specific fractures. External splintage is most useful in simple fractures of the long bones that result in minimal displacement. It can be appropriate, nevertheless, in severely comminuted fractures that are not amenable to simple repair with internal fixation. A proper splint should immobilize the joints proximal and distal to the fracture. Even pressure should be applied from the foot to the proximal end of the splint or cast; any ring of pressure may result in pendulous edema, avascular necrosis, and gangrene.

Aftercare is important to the success of splintage. The animal's owner must see to it that the splinting device remains dry and clean and does not wear excessively. Daily examination by the owner and proper medication of areas of the skin that are in contact with the end of the splint are essential. The feet or toes generally may be palpated through the tape or observed at deliberately exposed sites in the splintage. Any indication of edema or pain on palpation is cause for examination at the veterinary clinic. The clinician must provide client education on the care of splints and casts at home and should confirm the effectiveness of his instruction by regular examination of the splint.

TEMPORARY SPLINTS

The primary goal of emergency treatment is to preserve life by providing a clear airway, stopping hemorrhage, and supporting the cardiovascular system by treatment for shock. Definitive treatment of lesions of the musculoskeletal system may be delayed by extensive emergency treatment and evaluation of that treatment.

Injury to the musculoskeletal system should not be ignored during this treatment. A closed oblique fracture, if not immobilized, may penetrate the skin, rupture vessels, or sever a peripheral nerve. Periosteal stripping may delay bone healing. Temporary splintage stabilizes the fracture, prevents and lessens edema, and reduces the likelihood of self-induced trauma. Although not perfect, stabilization reduces periosteal stripping, hemorrhage, and subsequent injury to surrounding vessels and nerves. It also reduces pain and lessens the shock due to pain.

Temporary Immobilization at Home

Emergency care of the injured patient should begin at the scene of the accident.

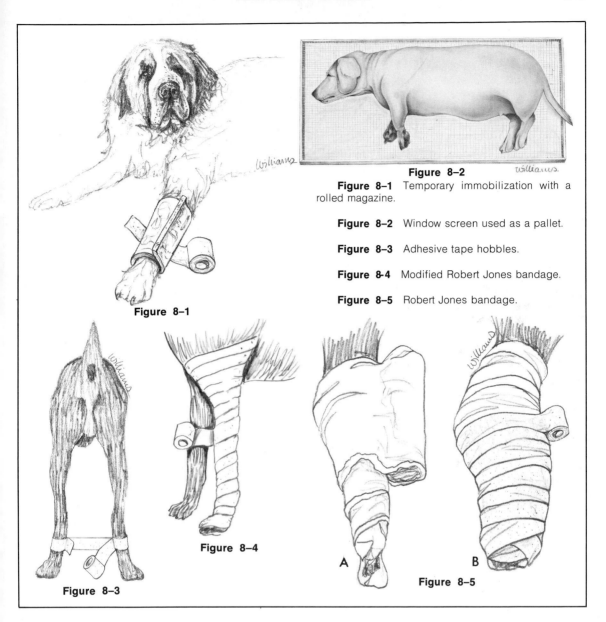

Figure 8–1

Figure 8–2

Figure 8–1 Temporary immobilization with a rolled magazine.

Figure 8–2 Window screen used as a pallet.

Figure 8–3 Adhesive tape hobbles.

Figure 8-4 Modified Robert Jones bandage.

Figure 8-5 Robert Jones bandage.

Figure 8–3

Figure 8–4

Figure 8–5

A   B

Transport to the veterinary hospital can be delayed for application of a pressure bandage to control superficial hemorrhage and a temporary dressing for immobilization of suspected limb fractures. The veterinarian or the receptionist should advise the owner of these steps. A simple clean bandage applied to an open fracture may be the first step to healing by preventing further contamination. The suspected forelimb fracture may be wrapped in a rolled magazine, bath towel, or roll cotton fixed with adhesive tape (Fig. 8–1).

Paraparesis following injury dictates that the animal should be placed on a blanket or pallet (Fig. 8–2) for transport and should not be lifted by the limbs or neck, nor should such animals with potential spinal fractures be handled carelessly by veterinary personnel; prevention of further trauma is an essential part of emergency care.

Tape Hobbles

Abduction of the rearlimbs in the dog and cat most often results from fractures of the pelvis or fracture-dislocation of the pubic symphysis and sacroiliac articulation. Adhesive tape may be applied to the hind limbs to prevent abduction (Fig. 8–3). Adhesive tape of sufficient size to cover at least one-half the length of the metatarsal bones is placed in stirrup fashion around the lateral metatarsus of one leg with tape applied to tape on the medial surface. The adhesive tape is extended to the other leg and is similarly applied so that the separation of the limbs approximately equals the distance between the greater trochanters. A ring of tape is contraindicated on the metatarsus since it might produce peripheral edema.

Fixation of a fractured limb to the other with tape is an alternative form of hobble recommended by some to prevent rotation, abduction, and adduction. The alternative hobble may be effective for protection of high femoral and humeral fractures, is especially useful in animals with short limbs, and can be applied in the presence of extensive soft tissue damage. The metacarpal or metatarsal area is padded with cast padding or dressing sponge covered with tape, leaving a tab for attachment to the opposite limb. When extensive instability exists, the padded metacarpal or metacarpal area may be bandaged together from the toes to the carpus or hocks.

Modified Robert Jones Bandage

The modified Robert Jones bandage is indicated when the prevention of edema is a primary concern and when stabilization of the fracture is of minimal concern. Salter type I and V fractures of the physis in the young may be temporarily splinted with well-padded bandages. Extensive wounds in the skin that prohibit adequate palpation may similarly be covered until radiographic examination is complete.

Cast padding is applied from the foot proximally to the upper humerus or femur (Fig. 8–4). The cast padding is overlapped 50 per cent as it is applied from the foot proximally and returned to the foot. The middle two toes should be exposed. The padding is covered with overlapping elastic adhesive tape from the distal to the proximal part of the limb. Two to 3 in. tape is indicated because 1 in. tape offers little stability.

Robert Jones Bandages

The Robert Jones bandage is the best temporary bandage for fractures of the limbs in small animals (Fig. 8–5). Although bulky, it both reduces and prevents edema. It tends to prevent further trauma caused by fractured fragments moving against soft tissues. It is indicated for all fractures of the limbs distal to the mid-shaft of the humerus and the femur in small animals. In proximal fractures in which the weight of the bandage is likely to cause angular displacement of the fracture, the bandage may be continued around the body and fixed with elastic tape or may be taped to the contralateral limb.

Application of the Robert Jones bandage is illustrated in Figures 8–44 to 8–49.

Temporary Coaptation and Traction Splints

Coaptation and traction splints may be applied for protection of the limb during emergency care and diagnosis. The former are applied closely to the shape of the limbs. A well-padded metal shoe (Figs. 8–10 to 8–13) is indicated for fractures of the bones distal to the elbow and the stifle. It offers little stability for fractures proximal to these joints.

The Schroeder-Thomas traction splint is demonstrated in Figures 8–111 to 8–134. In temporary application, the bones are fixed in a neutral position without attempts to reduce or align the fractures. The splint need not be accurately structured to conform to the shape of the limb; a straight rod cranial and caudal from the ring to the foot is acceptable for emergency support. The ring should be rotated inward under the axilla or pelvis to prevent outward pressure on the humerus or femur. Complete padding should be applied and immobilization should be insured to prevent pressure rings and irritation to the skin by adhesive tape. Although useful for temporary immobilization of fractures of the limb distal to the shoulder and femoral neck, a Schroeder-Thomas splint with extension of the elbow or stifle should not remain in place for more than three days.

Other Temporary Splints

Other splints and casts may be used for temporary immobilization. A shoulder sling (Figs. 8–148 to 8–153) is useful for fractures of the scapula and proximal humerus. Temporary stabilization of a limb may be achieved with Vet Set* applied as a channel for ease of application and removal or with a spica to cover the shoulder. Vertebral stability is easily achieved with a basswood or yucca board vertebral splint (Figs. 8–21 to 8–25).

COAPTATION SPLINTS

Since coaptation splints are made to resemble closely the shape of the limb, there is a marked similarity in the design of splints produced. The choice of splint material depends, therefore, on availability, the size of the animal, and personal perference. With these factors in mind, we will cover a wide variety of splint materials in the following pages.

Adhesive tape may be applied to the caudal and cranial surfaces of the foot, joined distal to the foot, and continued so as to attach the limb to the splint. A piece of adhesive tape may be spiralled around the cranial and caudal pieces to increase the fixation to the skin. A ring of tape should never be applied.

The hair of long-haired dogs should be removed by clipping and the limb should be washed and dried with alcohol or defatted with ether to increase the holding capacity of the adhesive tape. Skin wounds should be treated by proper cleansing and medication before the splint is applied. In general, the limb is padded and a suitable splint material is applied and fixed to the adhesive tape. The splint material is then covered with a bandage and taped. The foot always should be rotated medially as the splint is applied.

The limb is wrapped with an absorbent cotton or cast padding material from the toe to the proximal end of the splint. The splint material (such as a tongue depressor, metal shoe, or yucca board) is fixed in position over the padding with the distal end of the splint material extending to the end of the digits. The preplaced adhesive tape is reflected and attached to the splint material and the fracture is reduced. A bandage is applied under even pressure by means of roll gauze or some other appropriate elastic bandage material. The bandage is covered with adhesive tape.

In large and active animals, an aluminum rod stirrup should be applied to the distal end of the splint. The stirrup will prevent excessive wear to the splint and will protect against separation of the adhesive tape fixation to the splint material. The splint should be covered with a stockinette to prevent soiling as the animal is awakening from the anesthesia. The stockinette may be removed when the animal is to be released from the clinic. This simple procedure will make rebandaging before discharge unnecessary. Splints and casts should be applied as carefully as possible on the first application. Radiographic examination of the reduction is essential in good fracture management.

Among the materials available for coaptation splints are tongue depressors, metal shoes, yucca board, basswood, plywood, and fiberboard. Tongue depressors may be cut in length and width for small dogs. They should be well padded and placed on the caudal surface of the foot. Tongue depressor splints are useful for fixation of fractures of the digits, metacarpals, and metatarsals.

Metal shoes (Mason metasplint) are commercially available through supply houses. The shoe is a channeled aluminum splint with its distal end rounded for surface contact and conformity to the foot. Several sizes are available, as are extensions for the splints. The metal shoe should be widened or narrowed to closely approximate the shape of the padded limb. Metal shoe splints are useful for fractures of the distal radius and ulna, fracture dislocations of the carpus, and fractures of the metacarpal and metatarsal bones. Plastic spoon splints* are also available commercially. They are applied similarly to the metal shoe. In general, they are supplied with excess length, permitting shortening with a hack saw.

Yucca board, which is obtained from the yucca plant, is an extremely useful material, but it is subject to considerable variation in quality, depending on the source and on care in production. The advantages of the material are ease of cutting and shaping when wet and stability in the molded form when dry. Because the material may be shaped to nearly approximate the shape of

---

*Vet-Set is distributed by Veterinary Products Industries, Phoenix, Ariz.

*Plastic spoon splints are available from Edgewood Surgical Co., Indianapolis, Ind.

the limb, less pressure results at the points of limb enlargement. The primary disadvantage is the relative unavailability of uniform high quality materials. Yucca board splints may be used for the same fractures as the metal shoe.

Plastic splint material is available that may be molded and easily cut when warmed. It retains the desired configuration upon cooling. At least one source is currently available,* and another appears likely in the future.* Adequate protection of the limb during application of the molded plastic splint is essential. The splint should cover a limited area so that vaporization of moisture from the limb is possible. Retention of excessive moisture within the bandage and plastic splint has resulted in marked excoriation of the skin in some patients. Nevertheless, the possibilities of excellent fixation exist for fractures of the distal bones of the limbs.

*A plastic splint sold under the name Orthoplast is manufactured by Johnson and Johnson, New Brunswick, N.J.

*A plastic splint with the designation PXMD-5637 is manufactured by the Union Carbide Corporation, Bound Brook, N.J.

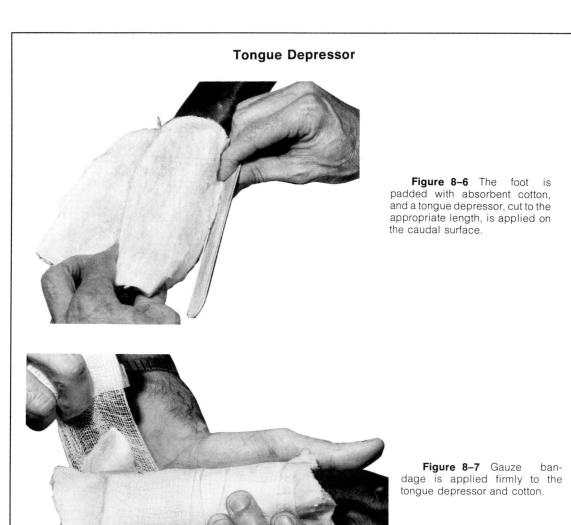

Tongue Depressor

Figure 8–6 The foot is padded with absorbent cotton, and a tongue depressor, cut to the appropriate length, is applied on the caudal surface.

Figure 8–7 Gauze bandage is applied firmly to the tongue depressor and cotton.

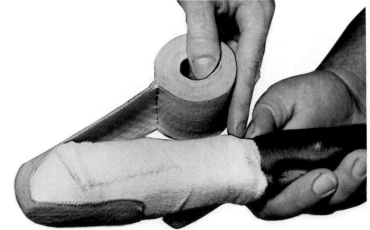

Figure 8–8 Overlapping tape is placed on the distal end of the splint.

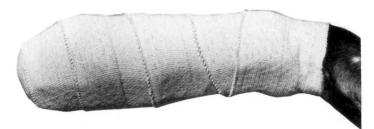

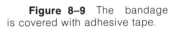

Figure 8–9 The bandage is covered with adhesive tape.

Metal Shoe

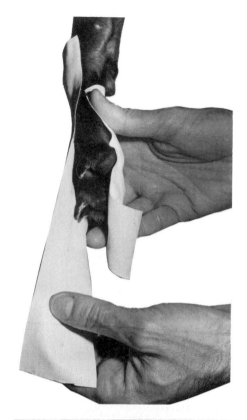

Figure 8–10 A strip of adhesive tape is applied to the caudal surface of the foot and is allowed to extend distal to the toes. A similar adhesive tape strip is applied to the cranial surface of the foot and extends beyond the strip applied to the caudal surface.

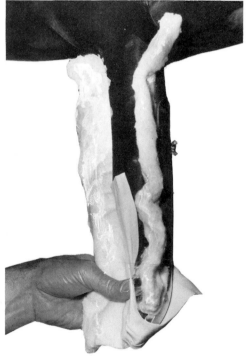

Figure 8–11 A suitable metal shoe is selected and is bent to fit the limb. The metal shoe should extend from the foot to the ventral aspect of the olecranon process. Absorbent cotton is rolled around the limb, and the metal shoe is applied on the caudal surface of the limb distal to the olecranon process.

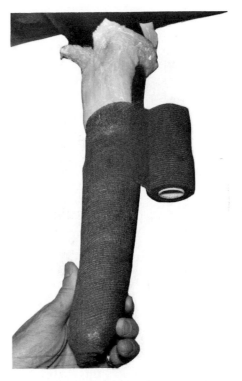

Figure 8–12 The adhesive tape is reflected caudally and is attached to the caudal surface of the metal shoe. Gauze or elastic bandage is applied from the foot to the proximal end of the splint.

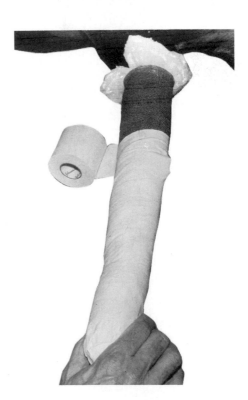

Figure 8–13 Adhesive tape is used to cover the bandage material.

Yucca Board

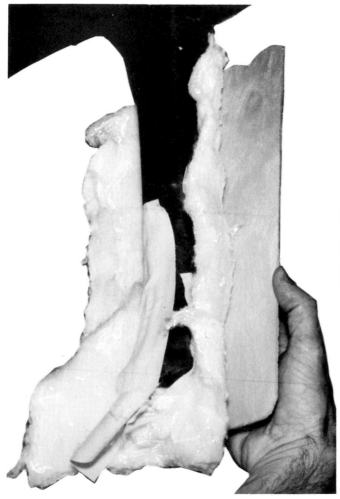

Figure 8–14 Adhesive tape is applied to the foot on the caudal and cranial surfaces with the cranial piece of adhesive tape extending beyond that on the caudal surface. The yucca board is wetted and cut to fit the limb, with the corners rounded and a small notch cut in the middle of the proximal end.

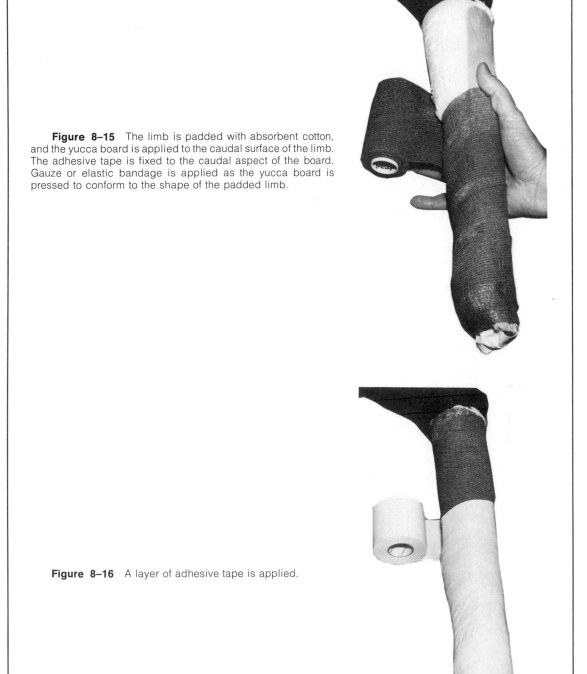

Figure 8–15 The limb is padded with absorbent cotton, and the yucca board is applied to the caudal surface of the limb. The adhesive tape is fixed to the caudal aspect of the board. Gauze or elastic bandage is applied as the yucca board is pressed to conform to the shape of the padded limb.

Figure 8–16 A layer of adhesive tape is applied.

Molded Plastic

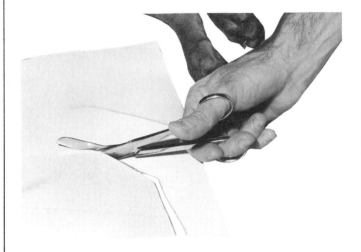

Figure 8–17 The plastic splint material is immersed in hot water until it becomes sufficiently pliable to be cut to the conformation desired and is applied over the padded limb.

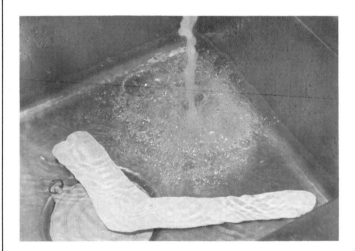

Figure 8–18 It may be softened and reshaped as required.

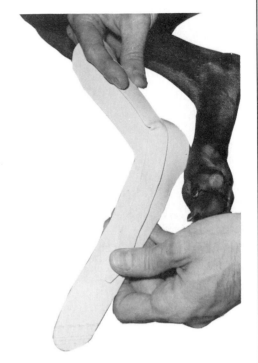

Figure 8–19 Additional support may be provided by the addition of heated strips of plastic to the outside surface of the splint.

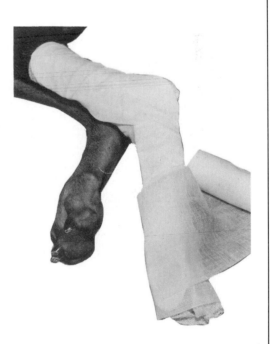

Figure 8–20 The plastic splint is covered with gauze or elastic bandage and tape. The material should not encircle the limb because of the likelihood of moisture entrapment.

Basswood Vertebral Splint

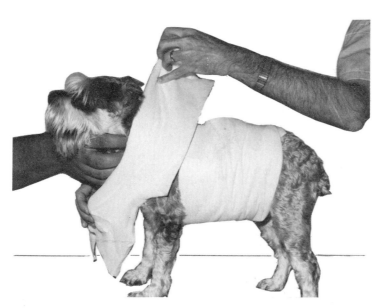

Figure 8–21 Basswood is used primarily as temporary splintage with heavy padding. It is most useful as a spinal or vertebral splint fixation for stability of the back. The animal's body is padded by abundant combine bandage that is cut to surround the limbs and pad the cervical region. The combine bandage is taped in place.

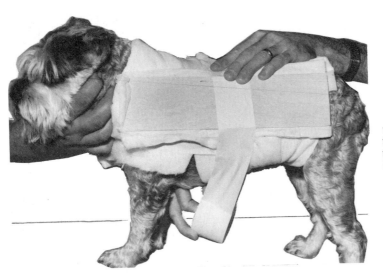

Figure 8–22 Strips of basswood are padded and applied on the caudolateral surfaces of the trunk from the cervical to the lower lumbar regions.

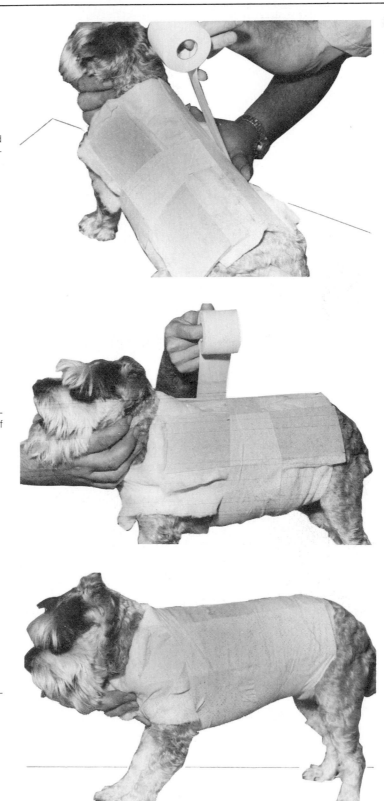

Figure 8–23 Yucca board may be used in place of the basswood.

Figure 8–24 Tape is applied to complete the fixation of the vertebrae.

Figure 8–25 The thoracolumbar vertebrae are immobile.

Plaster Cervical Vertebral Cast

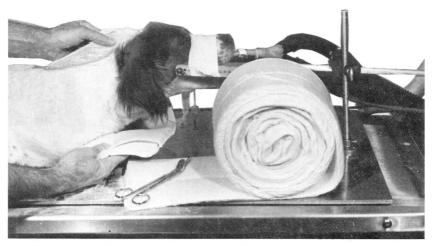

Figure 8–26   A combination plaster-padding roll is marketed commercially as Vet Set.* Several layers of plaster are covered with foam on the inside and cotton on the outside. The head and neck are stabilized, and a length of appropriate width plaster roll is cut to encircle the neck.

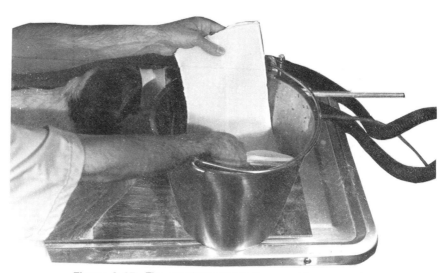

Figure 8–27   The cut plaster roll is immersed in warm water.

*Vet Set is distributed by Veterinary Products Industries, Phoenix, Ariz. It was previously distributed by Jensen-Salsbery Co. under the trade name Minute-On.

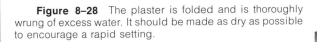

Figure 8–28 The plaster is folded and is thoroughly wrung of excess water. It should be made as dry as possible to encourage a rapid setting.

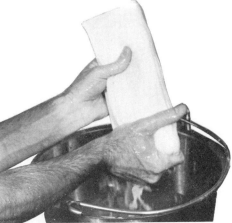

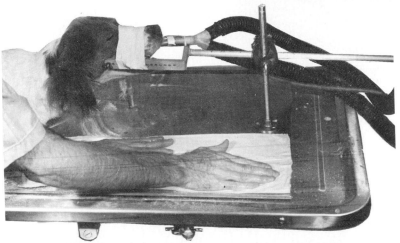

Figure 8–29 The plaster roll is smoothed on a flat surface.

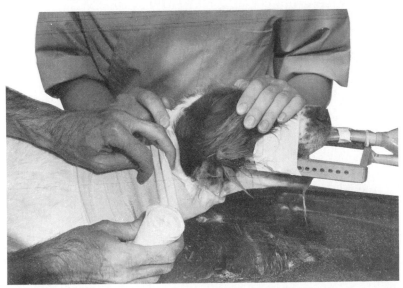

Figure 8–30 The plaster is positioned snugly on the neck and is covered with an elastic bandage. The foam-padded inner surface is rolled outward to relieve pressure behind the ears and at the points of the shoulders.

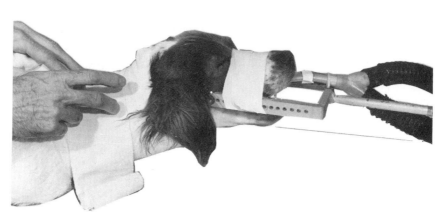

Figure 8–31   The plaster is allowed to set until firm.

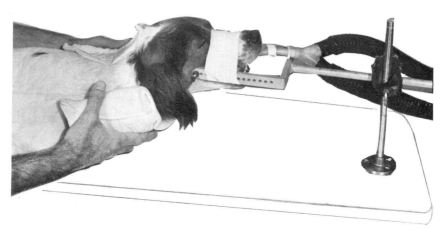

Figure 8–32   The plaster cast is opened by manual pressure to create a hinge opposite to the overlapping side.

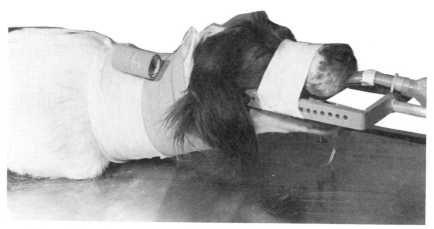

Figure 8–33   The plaster is reapplied and is firmly fixed with elastic gauze and tape or elastic tape alone.

Foam Rubber Cervical Splint

Figure 8–34 Foam rubber provides a light base for a cervical splint in cats and small dogs. A piece of ¾ to 1 inch thick foam rubber is cut to circle the neck and fit firmly between the head and the shoulders.

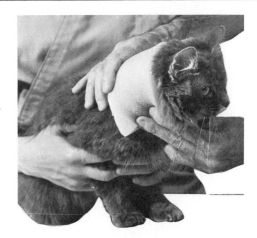

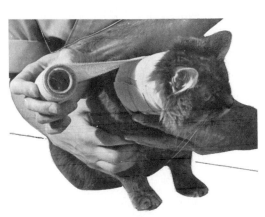

Figure 8–35 The foam rubber is wrapped firmly around the neck with elastic tape.

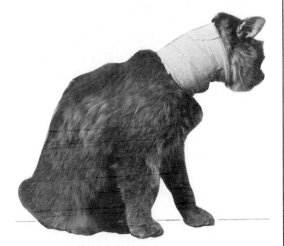

Figure 8–36 The splint affords stability with comfort and light weight.

Wire Frame Neck Brace

Figure 8–37 A wire frame neck brace is used by some clinicians. Suitable rings are fabricated for the cranial and caudal cervical regions and are joined by adjustable rods. The rings are padded, and the device is fixed with tape to a halter or to fixation tape on the thorax.

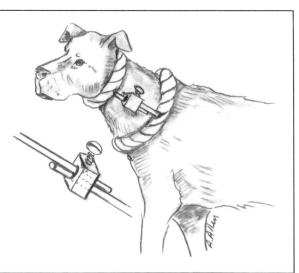

Plywood or Fiberboard

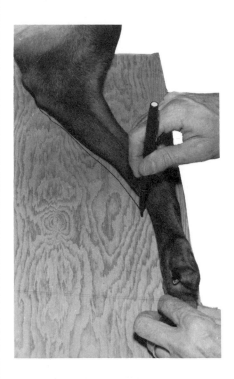

Figure 8–38 Plywood coaptation splints are useful for fixation of fractures of the tibia and fracture-dislocations of the hock. The normal limb is placed on a suitable plywood board and outlined with a felt marker.

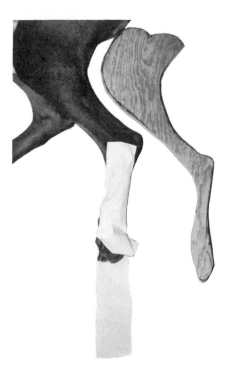

Figure 8–39 A saw is used to cut the plywood in silhouette form with a notch on the proximal end in the region of the thigh. Adhesive tape is placed on the lateral and medial surfaces of the foot, with the longer piece secured on the medial surface.

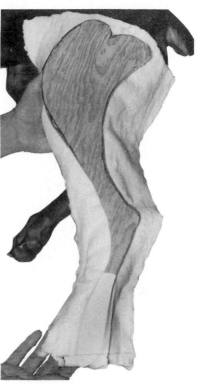

Figure 8–40 The limb is padded with full thickness roll absorbent cotton. The plywood is applied to the lateral surface of the limb, and the adhesive tape is fixed to the lateral surface of the distal end of the plywood.

Figure 8–41 Elastic gauze is applied over the plywood splint and adjacent padding. The gauze may be passed through the notch at the proximal end of the splint for proper fixation.

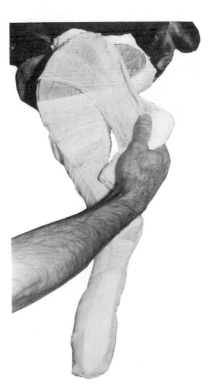

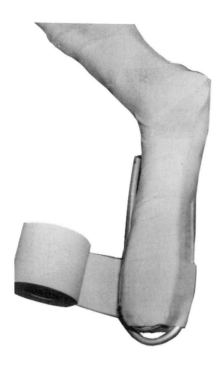

Figure 8–42 An aluminum stirrup is then placed on the distal end.

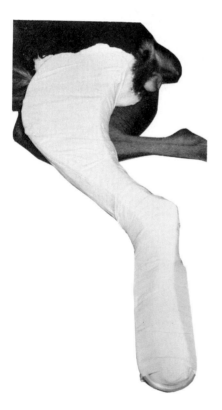

Figure 8–43 The splint is covered with adhesive tape.

Basswood can neither be bent nor easily cut. It is primarily used as temporary splintage or for rigid immobilization of the spine by whole body splintage.

Plywood or fiberboard is abundantly available through lumber supply houses. The board may be marked and cut to the shape of the limb with a band saw or a coping saw. Plywood in ⅛ in. to ¼ in. thickness or standard fiberboard may be placed adjacent to the limb with abundant padding. Board splints are effective for fractures of the tibia and immobilization of the hock.

ROBERT JONES BANDAGE

The Robert Jones bandage is a dressing that immobilizes the limb and applies even pressure, thereby preventing or reducing edema. Although used primarily in the treatment of severely traumatized limbs, it is the best single dressing for the temporary immobilization of limbs. It can be applied with relative ease from commonly available materials and provides an excellent form of immobilization while preventing edema and secondary complications that frequently arise following disruption of bone and soft tissues.

Application

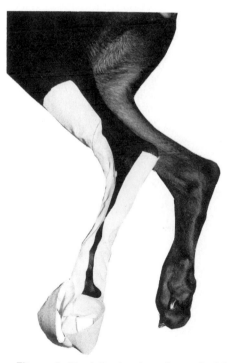

Figure 8–44 Adhesive tape is applied to the cranial and caudal surfaces of the lower limb and is extended distal to the foot. The adhesive tape should be lightly joined and rolled outward so that it may be separated.

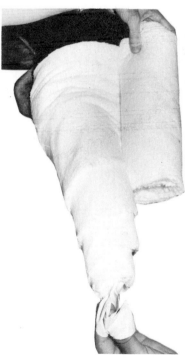

Figure 8–45 The limb is tightly rolled with absorbent cotton. The paper filler in the cotton roll has been removed and the cotton has been rewound.

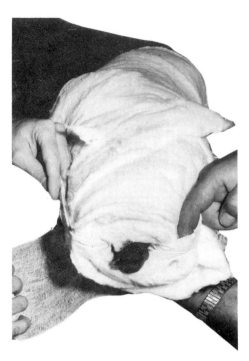

Figure 8–46 Two or more pounds of cotton may be applied to an average limb until a large bulk of padding is in place. The tape is reflected on the outside of the cotton, and the third and fourth digits are left exposed.

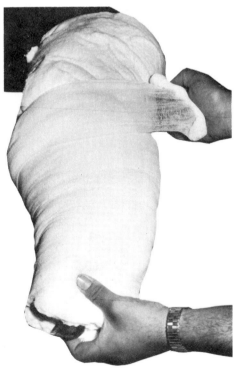

Figure 8–47 The absorbent cotton is tightly covered with elastic gauze (Vetrap, Kling, Coban).

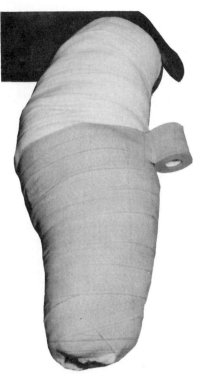

Figure 8–48 Elastic tape is applied over the gauze dressing. Tension is used during application so that a firm finished bandage is achieved.

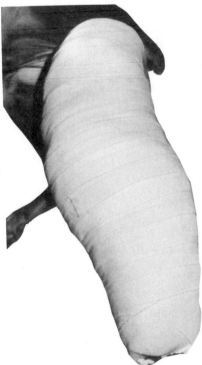

Figure 8–49 Circulation to the toes may be evaluated in the exposed digits. In fractures of the proximal femur or humerus, padding, elastic gauze, and elastic tape may be extended proximally to encircle the body.

PLASTER OF PARIS SPLINTS

Plaster of Paris is manufactured from solid crystalline gypsum or calcium sulfate dihydrate. The plaster material is pulverized and subjected to high temperatures to drive out the water of crystallization. The hardening of the plaster is then brought about by the addition of water. The setting time of plaster is measured from the time the plaster is wet to the time at which the cast becomes firm. Setting time is controlled by the type of plaster, the wetness of the plaster, and the extent to which the plaster is wrung after wetting. Fast-setting plaster becomes firm within five to eight minutes;* "extra-fast-setting" plaster will become firm in two to four minutes.† Water must vaporize from the surface before the cast gains maximum strength (four to six hours). Resin plasters are stronger than ordinary plaster of Paris. Their additional strength provides a stronger but lighter cast.

The equipment needed for plaster casts includes plaster of Paris in roll form (2 in. and 3 in. wide), cast padding, stockinette, adhesive tape, and plaster of Paris in splint form.‡ The latter form is more heavily impregnated with plaster of Paris and serves to provide additional strength in regions where bending is likely.

The animal should be given general anesthesia to allow proper reduction of the fracture and to complete immobilization while the plaster is setting. It may be helpful to suspend the limb from an intravenous stand by a rope or adhesive tape attached to the foot. Such a position will allow the weight of the animal to distract the joints of the limb and assist in positioning the fractured fragments. The same results may be achieved by positioning ropes around the attachment of the limb to the body and foot or by manipulation by an assistant. The presence of an assistant allows the clinician to apply the splint with the limb in a horizontal position.

A used piece of disposable draping material may be placed over the body to prevent soiling the hair with plaster. The limb can be exposed through a hole in the drape. Tapes applied to the foot are incorporated in the plaster of Paris splint. In most instances, the third and fourth digits are allowed to remain exposed so that the limb may be checked for edema or signs of inflammation. Casts applied to the forelimbs generally should extend well into the humeral area; those applied to the rearlimbs should extend into the femoral area. Only enough plaster of Paris should be applied to support the weight and activity of the animal. The use of plaster splints to increase strength without appreciably increasing weight is recommended. Plaster is easy to use and will remain moistened during application. Should it be wrung too dry, it may be remoistened during application. A small amount of water may be used to smooth the finished cast.

The limb should be well padded with cast padding before the plaster is applied. A double layer of padding is used, with four layers being placed over the pressure points. Incorporation of a saw of Gigli wire is generally not recommended because the moisture in the cast will rust the wire saw; deterioration of the metal will cause it to break when needed for cast removal. When the plaster of Paris is dry, a layer of stockinette is placed over the cast and is taped at the top and bottom. This stockinette will prevent soiling with urine or feces while the animal is awakening. When the animal is discharged, the accessory layer of stockinette may be removed and the animal may be released with a clean cast.

The cast should be rechecked for comfort, stability, and the absence of swelling 24 hours after application. Radiographic evaluation at this time is advisable. The cast should be rechecked in one week and every two or three weeks thereafter until it is removed. The owner should be requested to examine the cast daily. Plaster of Paris casts must be kept dry. As with other splints, an aluminum stirrup placed at the distal end will reduce the amount of damage to the plaster caused by walking.

Removal of the plaster of Paris cast is best done with a cast cutter (vibrating saw) and a cast spreader. The animal should be anesthetized and the cast should be cut with the vibrating saw. It may be separated at the cut, and the underlying padding and stockinette can be severed with scissors. The

---

*Zoroc Resin Plaster Bandage is manufactured by Johnson and Johnson, New Brunswick, N.J.

†Specialist Ultra Fast Setting Plaster Bandage is manufactured by Johnson and Johnson, New Brunswick, N.J.

‡Specialist Plaster Splint is manufactured by Johnson and Johnson, New Brunswick, N.J.

difficulty of removal without a cast cutter has caused some clinicians to utilize a split cast. The split cast is an unpadded plaster of Paris cast that can be removed and replaced as needed. It is a functional cast for use when re-evaluation of the limb is advisable, but it cannot be structured with the strength of the standard plaster of Paris cast and is generally unacceptable in heavier dogs.

Plaster of Paris splints are useful as coaptation devices; they allow close positioning of the fractured fragments. Plaster of Paris splintage is particularly useful in fractures of the radius and ulna and of the tibia; they have little value for fractures of the femur or the humerus unless a body spica is used. Spicas are cumbersome and generally are not used in small animals. The surgeon should manipulate the limb before applying a cast to be sure that reduction of the fracture is possible by a closed approach.

In recent years, modification of standard plaster has been achieved. A prefabricated multilayered plaster covered with cotton and foam rubber is marketed under the trade name of Vet Set.* A knitted polyester and cotton fabric has also been produced with polyurethane that is water-activated.† This preparation is lightweight and sets in seven minutes. It lacks the strength of plaster but has found use in small and large animal casts.

*Vet Set was previously marketed as Minute-On by Jensen-Salsbery Co. It is now distributed by Veterinary Products Industries, Phoenix, Ariz.

†Cutter Biomedical, Division of Cutter Laboratories, Inc., San Diego, Cal. 92111.

Forelimb Cast

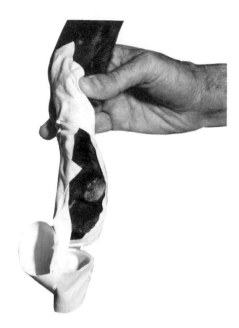

Figure 8–50 Strips of adhesive tape are placed on the cranial and caudal surfaces of the foot and are allowed to protrude several inches distal to the end. A spiral tape may be applied for added fixation. The tapes may be applied to opposite sides of a tongue depressor to facilitate removal.

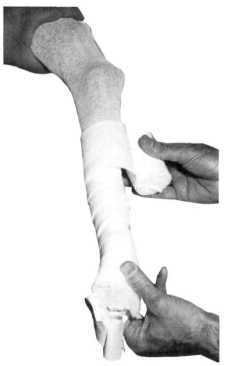

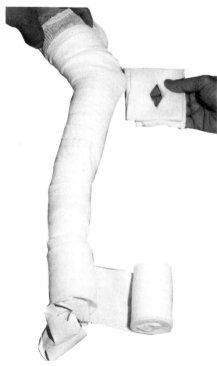

Figure 8–51 An orthopedic stockinette is applied to the limb with extra length at top and bottom. The fracture or dislocation is reduced, and the cast padding is applied in double thickness.

Figure 8–52 The padding may be overlapped as it is applied to the limb from the foot upward and then overlapped as it is returned to the foot. The olecranon is doubly padded with cast padding.

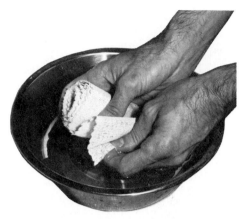

Figure 8–53 Plaster of Paris is wetted by immersion in water until the bubbles stop (5 to 10 seconds). The end is grasped in one hand.

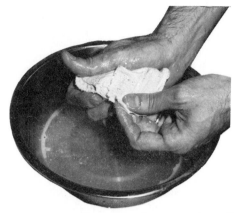

Figure 8–54 The water is wrung from the plaster.

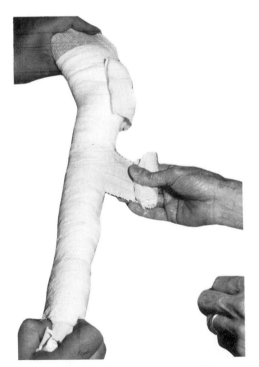

Figure 8–55 Plaster of Paris is rolled onto the limb from the distal to the proximal portion and is returned distally. The third and fourth digits should remain exposed.

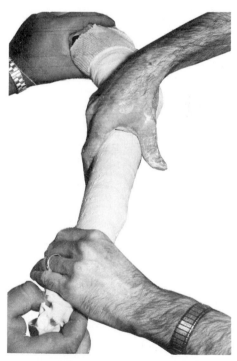

Figure 8–56 The limb is readjusted to assure proper reduction of the fracture or dislocation.

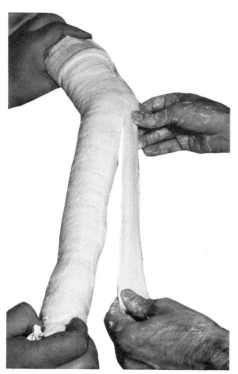

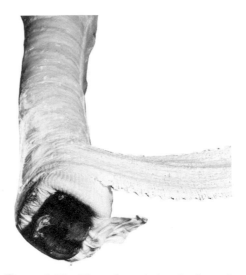

Figure 8–58 When the plaster is firm, the stockinette and tape on the distal end are reflected proximally and are fixed in place with a single strip of plaster splint.

Figure 8–57 Plaster splints may be applied on the cranial and caudal surfaces of the cast to add strength.

Figure 8–59 The plaster splint is similarly used to fix the distally reflected stockinette on the proximal end of the cast. A final roll of plaster may be applied and smoothed in place. Rubber gloves may be worn to help smooth the cast; at no time should finger pressure be allowed to indent the plaster.

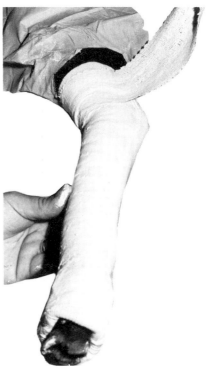

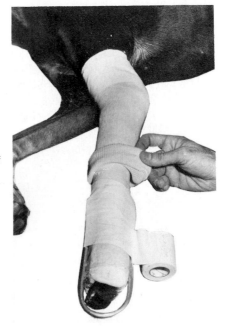

Figure 8–60 A metal stirrup is taped to the distal end of the cast.

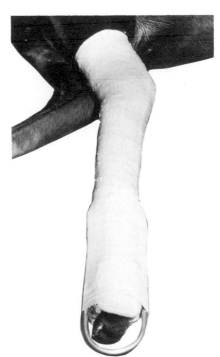

Figure 8–61 The stockinette is applied temporarily and is removed when the animal is discharged from the clinic.

Rearlimb Cast

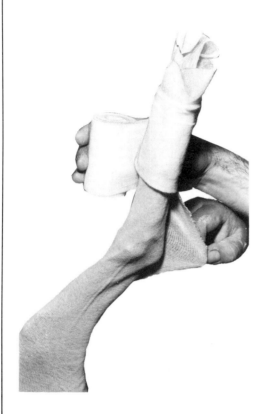

Figure 8–62 After taping the foot as in the fore-limb cast, the clinician applies an orthopedic stockinette to the limb and leaves extra length at the top and bottom. The fracture or dislocation is reduced and cast padding is applied.

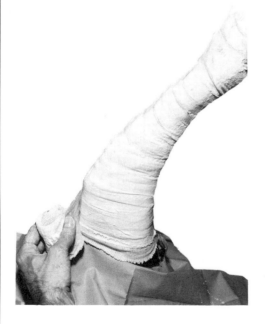

Figure 8–63 After the tuber calcanei is doubly padded with cast padding, plaster of Paris is wetted and rolled onto the limb from the distal portion to the proximal end and is returned distally. The third and fourth digits should remain exposed.

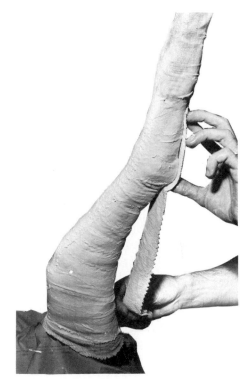

Figure 8–64 Plaster strips may be applied on the cranial and caudal surfaces of the cast to add strength. The limb is readjusted with palm pressure to assure proper reduction of the fracture or dislocation.

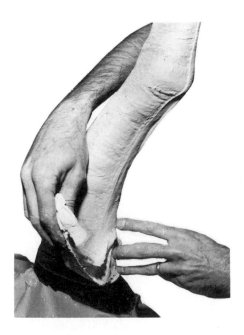

Figure 8–65 When the plaster is firm, the stockinette on the proximal end is reflected distally and fixed in place with a single strip of plaster splint.

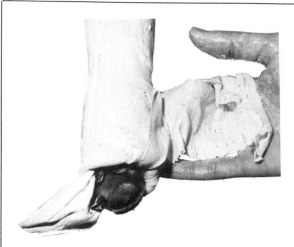

Figure 8–66 The stockinette and tape at the distal end are reflected and are fixed with a plaster splint. A final roll of plaster may be applied and smoothed in place.

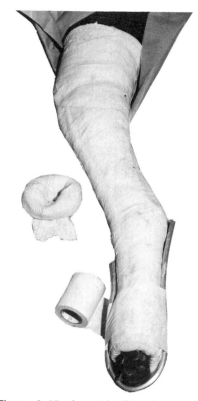

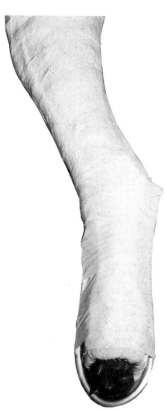

Figure 8–67 A metal stirrup is taped to the distal end of the cast.

Figure 8–68 The stockinette is applied temporarily and is removed when the animal is discharged.

Suspension of the limb by means of an intravenous stand lessens the tension around the thigh muscles. The horizontally applied cast should be firmly tightened in the region of these muscles or it will be loose when the animal awakens.

Removing the Cast

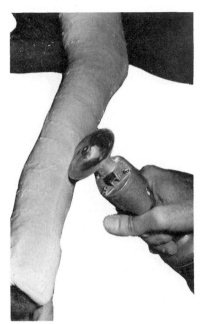

Figure 8–69 The plaster is cut longitudinally on the lateral side (and on the medial side if necessary). Care is taken not to traumatize the skin.

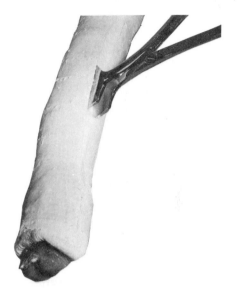

Figure 8–70 The plaster is separated with cast spreaders.

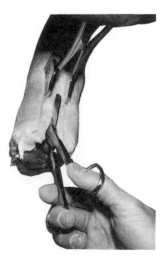

Figure 8–71 The cast padding and stockinette are cut with scissors.

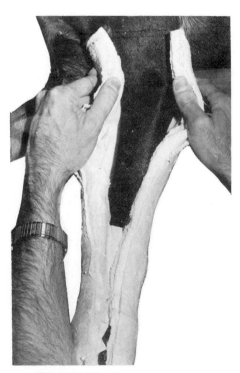

Figure 8–72 The cast is removed.

Split Cast

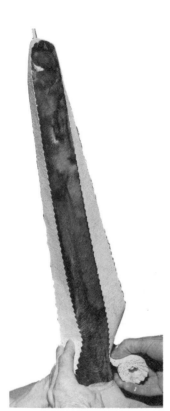

Figure 8–73 With the limb suspended and the bones properly positioned, plaster of Paris is unrolled to cover the cranial and caudal aspects of the limb.

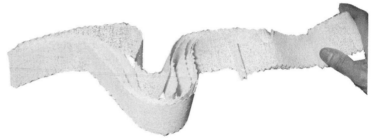

Figure 8–74 The measured plaster roll is doubled four or five times so that multiple layers of plaster are present. The approximate midpoint of the plaster is notched with scissors.

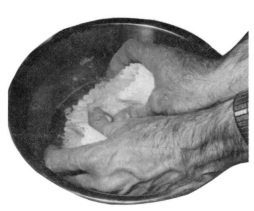

Figure 8–75 Each end is rolled toward the center, and the plaster is submerged in warm water.

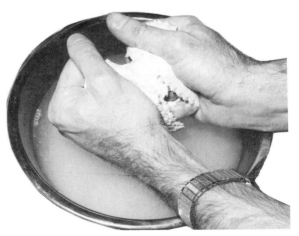

Figure 8–76 The water is squeezed from the plaster strips.

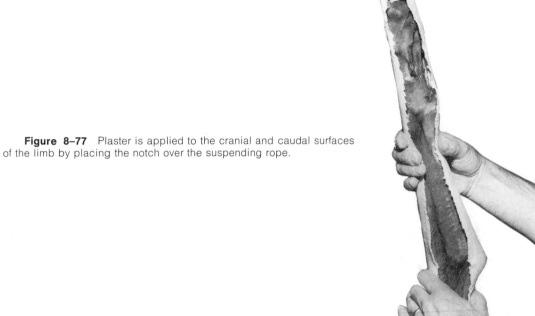

Figure 8–77 Plaster is applied to the cranial and caudal surfaces of the limb by placing the notch over the suspending rope.

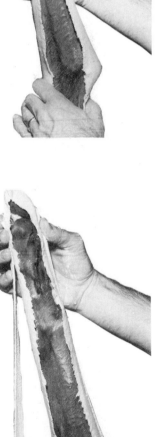

Figure 8–78 Additional plaster splints may be applied for greater strength.

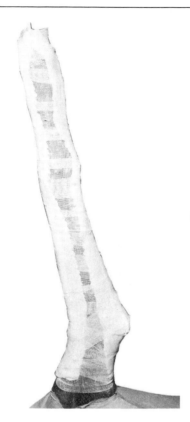

Figure 8–79 The plaster is smoothed and is loosely fixed in place with a roll of gauze bandage.

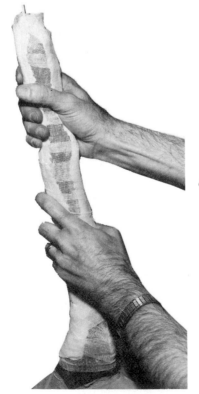

Figure 8–80 All edges should be rounded as the fracture is reduced.

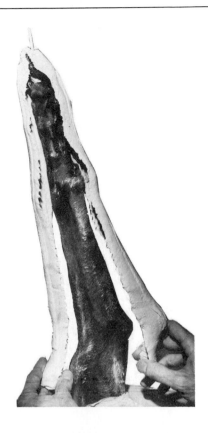

Figure 8–81 When the plaster has dried, the gauze is removed, the notched portion is severed with scissors, and the cast is removed from the limb.

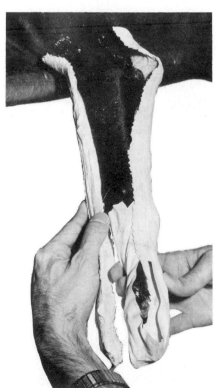

Figure 8–82 The suspending rope is removed, the fracture or dislocation is repositioned, and the split cast is reapplied by attachment of tape to the foot.

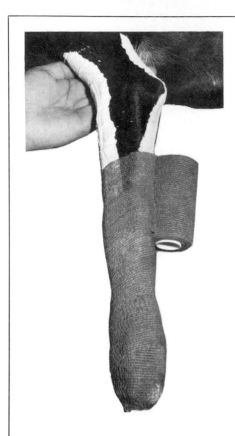

Figure 8–83   Gauze or an elastic bandage is applied.

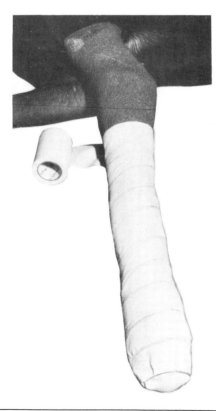

Figure 8–84   The bandage is covered with adhesive tape; a stirrup may be applied.

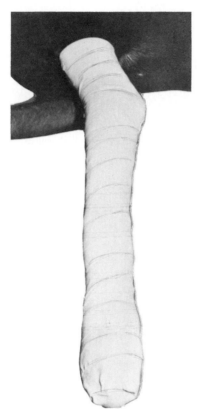

Figure 8–85   The split case is most applicable to fractures and dislocations of the forelimb rather than the heavily muscled rearlimb.

Fabricated Plaster Channel Splint

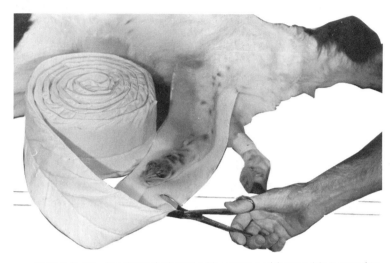

Figure 8–86 Fabricated plaster with cotton and foam rubber covering (Vet Set) may be applied as a channel lower limb cast or as a spica. The fabricated plaster roll is cut to fit the length of the forelimb from available widths.

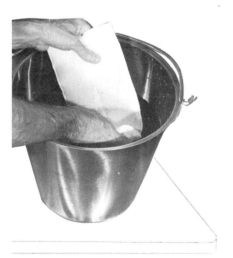

Figure 8–87 The plaster roll is immersed in water.

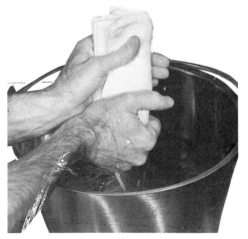

Figure 8–88 The plaster is folded and wrung dry.

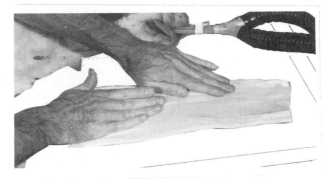

Figure 8–89 The plaster roll is smoothed on a flat surface.

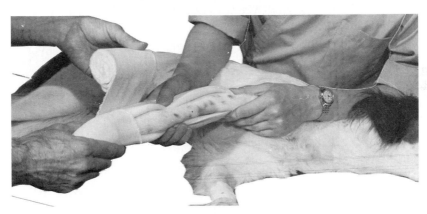

Figure 8–90 The plaster is applied to the caudal surface of the forelimb with the foam side toward the skin. The edges are folded back to reduce sharp edges, and an elastic bandage is applied.

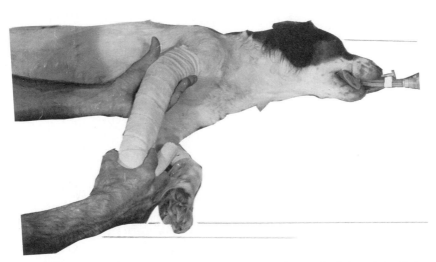

Figure 8–91 Alignment of the limb is achieved by manipulation of the limb through the plaster. The palms and proximal fingers are used for manipulation to prevent finger indentations of the cast.

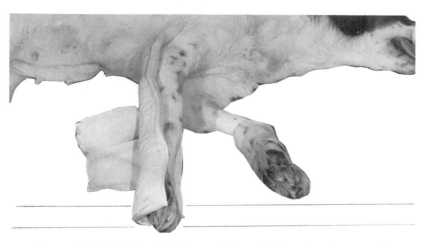

Figure 8–92   After the plaster has set, the elastic bandage is removed.

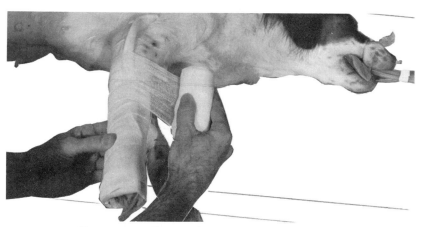

Figure 8–93   The cast is covered with elastic gauze.

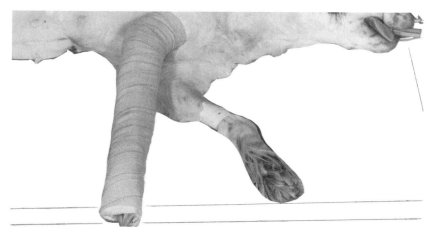

Figure 8–94   A final layer of elastic tape is applied.

Plaster Spica

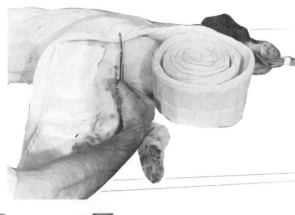

Figure 8–95 A length of appropriate width fabricated plaster (Vet Set) is cut to cover the medial side of the lower limb and the lateral side of the limb to the dorsal scapular border.

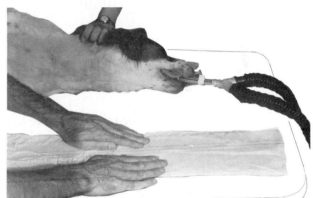

Figure 8–96 The plaster is immersed in warm water and wrung dry. The plaster is smoothed on a flat surface.

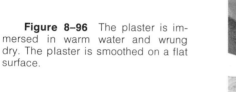

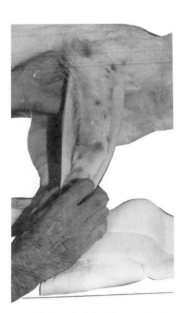

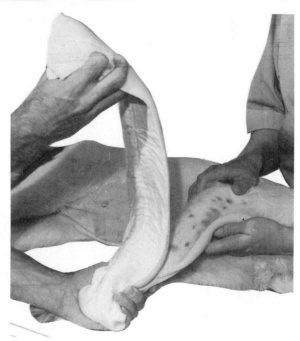

Figure 8–97 The plaster is applied on the medial side of the forelimb from the elbow to the foot.

Figure 8–98 The remainder is folded over the end of the foot and proximally on the lateral side of the limb and shoulder.

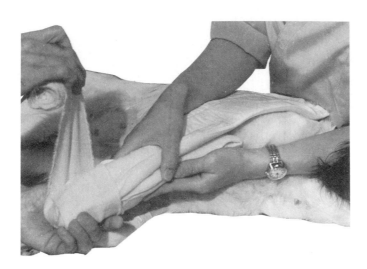

Figure 8–99 The edges of the plaster and foam rubber are folded outward to lessen sharp edges, and the cast is wrapped with an elastic bandage.

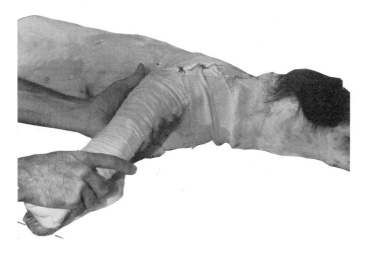

Figure 8–100 The elastic bandage is wrapped around the trunk to hold the plaster against the skin, and the limb is manipulated to align the bones.

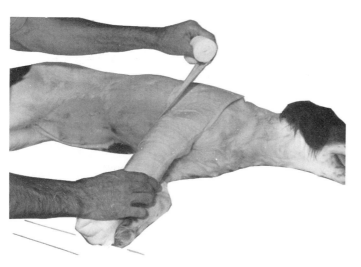

Figure 8–101 When the plaster has set, the elastic bandage is removed and is replaced with elastic gauze.

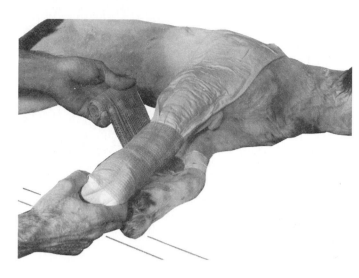

Figure 8–102 Additional strength may be provided by wrapping the cast with water-activated polyurethane instead of elastic gauze.

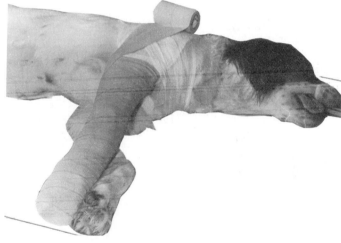

Figure 8–103 The elastic gauze is wrapped around the upper plaster and the trunk and is covered with elastic tape.

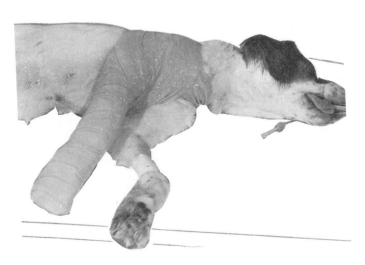

Figure 8–104 The cast is lightweight and provides adequate support for the upper limb. Traction is not provided.

CASTING TAPES

Several suppliers offer casting materials other than plaster. The most commonly used are activated by water. Hexcelite* is a polypropylene orthopedic tape that sets in approximately three to five minutes. It is lightweight and can be cut with bandage scissors or a cast saw. Cuttercast casting tape* is a polyester and cotton knitted fabric that has been impregnated with a water-activated polyurethane. The lightweight cast sets in approximately seven minutes and can bear weight 15 minutes later. The latter will be demonstrated.

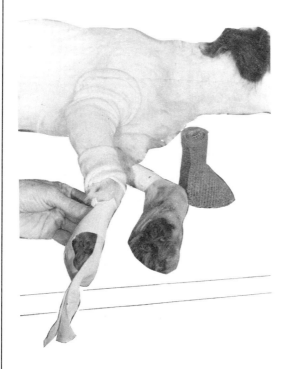

Figure 8–105 Adhesive tape is applied to the front and back of the foot and is fixed with a spiral of tape. The ends of the tape are applied to opposite sides of a tongue depressor. The limb is covered with a single-layer synthetic stockinette.

*Hexcelite Orthopedic Tape, Hexcel Medical Products, Dublin, CA 94566.

*Cuttercast Casting Tape, Cutter Biomedical, Division of Cutter Laboratories, Inc., San Diego, CA 94111.

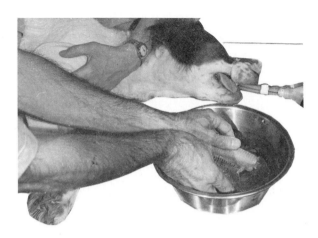

Figure 8–106 The Cuttercast is immersed in room temperature water. Hot water may result in excessive exothermic reaction.

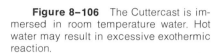

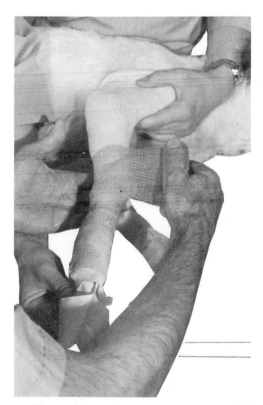

Figure 8–107 The casting tape is applied over a synthetic stockinette without cotton padding. Wet cotton padding or wet stockinette may cause a skin reaction.

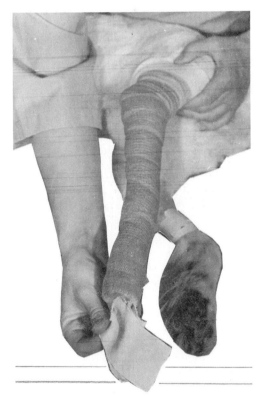

Figure 8–108 The casting tape is overlapped and is applied with even pressure. The limb is manipulated and is held as the casting tape sets. Skin irritation may result in certain individuals. Plastic gloves may be used during application in those with sensitivity.

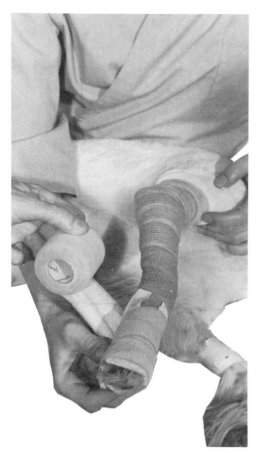

Figure 8–109 The stockinette and tape over the foot are retracted proximally and are fixed with porous elastic tape to expose the third and fourth toes.

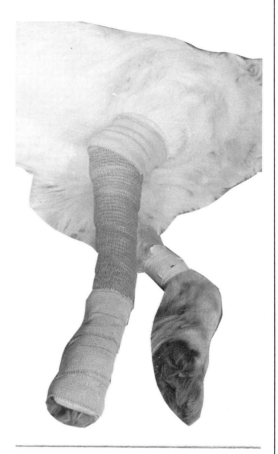

Figure 8–110 The stockinette at the proximal end of the cast is reflected distally and is fixed with elastic adhesive tape. The cast may be removed with a cast cutter, cast scissors, or by unwrapping the tape.

SCHROEDER-THOMAS SPLINTS

The Thomas splint is a walking splint designed with a ring circling the limb attachment (inguinal or pectoral) and rods projecting to the bottom of the foot. A Schroeder or modified Thomas splint is altered in configuration to fit the shape of the animal's limb and the type of fracture. Schroeder-Thomas splints may be used to reduce and fix appropriate fractures of any of the bones of the limbs from the humerus and femur to the metacarpals and metatarsals.

The materials for construction include aluminum splint rod, Johnson and Johnson combine bandage, cotton, and adhesive tape. The aluminum splint rod is available in 6 ft. lengths with diameters of $\frac{1}{8}$ in., $\frac{3}{16}$ in., and $\frac{3}{8}$ in. A set of wooden ring blocks and a vise are useful in shaping the splints. The aluminum rod may be cut with bolt cutters or sawed with a hack saw.

Although the Schroeder-Thomas splint consists of a padded elliptical ring and angled rods that join distally, the exact shape will depend upon the fractured bone. If one remembers that tension must be applied to separate the joints at each end of the fractured bone, the scheme for splint construction will be more apparent. Tensions applied in the correct direction allow the fractured fragments to be separated and aligned. The splint, as constructed for fractures of the radius and ulna, should be nearly straight, whereas a bend of 90° is recommended for repair of the humerus. Similarly, the configuration in the rearlimb is different for femoral and tibial fractures. The caudal wire in each fracture is straight. In fractures of the femur, the bend at the stifle is placed ventrally so that tension may be applied to the tibia, separating the fractured femoral fragments. The bend for tibial fractures is more proximal so that tension may be drawn on the femur, thus distracting fragments in the tibia.

The elliptical ring at the top of the modified Thomas splint should closely approximate the size of the limb at the body. An excessively large ring will permit slippage and the accumulation of debris; too small a ring will result in edema. Rubber rings made to fit the ring block are useful in determining proper size. The ring should be oval to correspond to the limb cross-section. The ring should be bent medially on its cranial and caudal aspects rather than being allowed to remain parallel to the upright rods in the splint. This medial deviation is necessary to conform to the angle of departure of the limb from the body. Similarly, the ventral portion of the ring should be bent further medially so that it curves slightly beneath the animal. This point of support should be ventral to the sternum in the forelimbs and slightly ventrolateral to the pelvic symphysis in the rearlimbs. The ring itself should not be overly padded, because such padding may cause undue pressure at the junction of the limb and the body.

As has been mentioned, tension is applied on the limb so as to facilitate separation of the joint on the extremities of the fractured bone. Combine roll is an excellent material for this task because it is soft and has sufficient strength to allow application of tension on the adjacent musculature. Other materials, such as gauze or tape, cannot be applied under as much tension without causing necrosis or edema. In fractures of the limbs, the portion of the combine roll that is attached to the foot is tightened first. The combine roll is then placed, and the portion covering the nonfractured segment is tightened. A fracture of the humerus would be repaired by preplacing combine roll and tightening the portion that encircles the radius and ulna. Similarly, with fractures of the tibia, the combine roll encircling the femur would be tightened following attachment to the foot. The combined roll that covers the fractured bone would be apposed and fixed with minimal tension. The primary purposes of the combine roll in the latter area are to reduce motion and to maintain even pressure on the limb.

It is apparent that a proper Thomas splint should consist of more than a few pieces of tape and an aluminum splint rod. The finished splint should be covered with adhesive tape; the latter should be applied as smoothly as possible. Where angles are turned, a small flap of tape may be left and cut and the ends overlapped. The general impression of a properly repaired fracture improves the attitude of the owner toward splint care. An aluminum stirrup is applied to the distal end of the splint. The stirrup, a simple U-shaped form, should cover the tape from the foot to the splint rod. The stirrup, which is essential to continued usefulness, is then itself taped. A stockinette is applied and is temporarily taped to the splint. The stockinette serves the same purpose for the splint as for plaster casts — namely, to prevent soiling by excrement while the animal is awakening from anesthesia and until the time of discharge. When the animal is ready for discharge, the stockinette is removed to display a clean splint.

If good aftercare is important in plaster casts, it is essential in modified Thomas splintage. The splint must remain dry and clean. The underside of the ring must be powdered daily; the limb must be palpated through the tape, particularly in the region of the hock and carpus, for signs of edema or pain. Client education and the opportunity to return the animal at any time are essential to good splint management. The splint is normally re-examined approximately ten days postoperatively and again three weeks later. In rapidly growing dogs, a more frequent examination may be necessary.

Rearlimb Schroeder-Thomas Splint

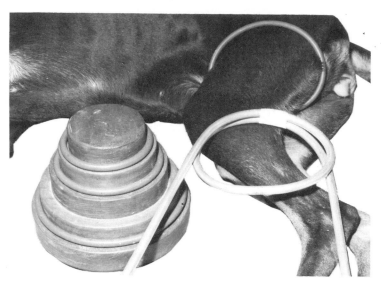

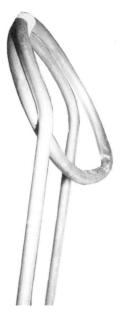

Figure 8–111 A ring is measured to fit the thigh. Rings of rubber on a wooden block of rings facilitate accurate measurement.

Figure 8–112 The ring should be oval and bent toward the animal's body on the ventral aspect.

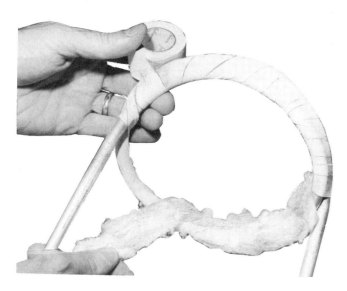

Figure 8–113 Tape is applied adhesive side out on the ventral portion of the ring; cotton is applied for padding, and the entire ring is covered with adhesive tape (applied as usual).

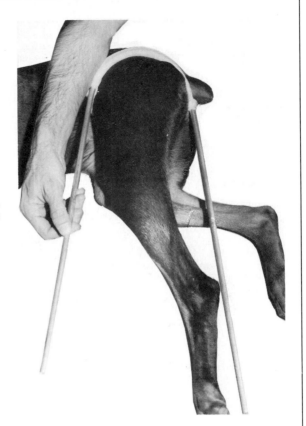

Figure 8–114 The vertical splint rod is measured to the end of the animal's foot and is shaped for the fracture.

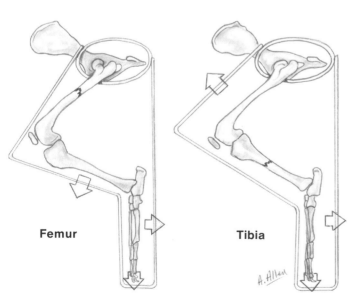

Femur

Tibia

Figure 8–115 Splints for fractures of the femur and the tibia should be formed as shown in the diagram.

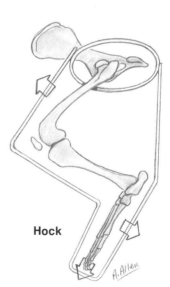

Hock

Figure 8–116 A modification of splint design for fracture-dislocation of the hock.

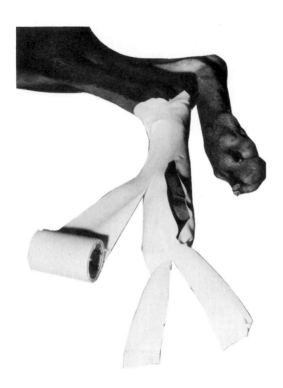

Figure 8–117 Strips of adhesive tape placed on the cranial and caudal surfaces of the foot are joined distal to the foot and are cut longitudinally. A spiral of tape may be applied for additional support.

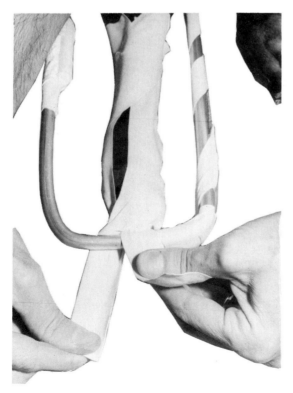

Figure 8–118 The surgeon applies fixation tape to the distal splint rod, rotating the lateral tape medially and the medial tape laterally to achieve inward rotation of the foot.

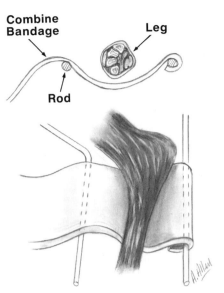

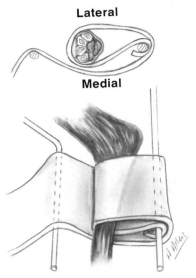

Figure 8–119 Combine roll is applied beneath the limb with the short end in the direction of pull.

Figure 8–120 The combine roll is wrapped around the leg and splint and then passed between the leg and the splint rod, where it is fixed.

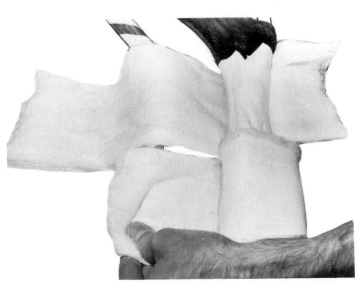

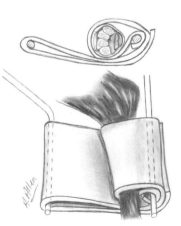

Figure 8–121 The combine roll is applied to the foot.

Figure 8–122 The bandage is wrapped firmly and is taped in place.

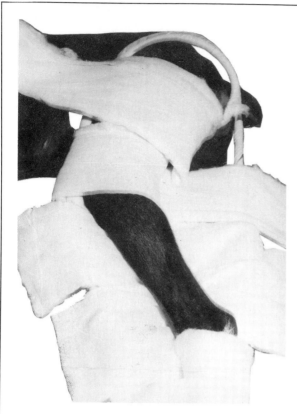

Figure 8–123 Combine roll is applied proximally and is tightened at the nonfractured bone (the femur).

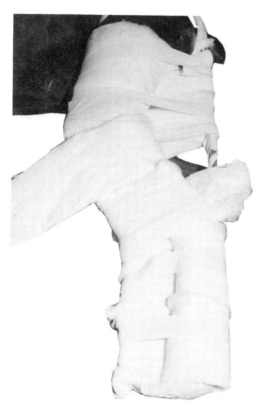

Figure 8–124 Combine bandage is loosely fixed in the region of the fractured tibia.

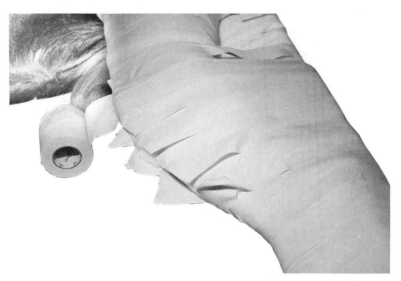

Figure 8–125 A smooth coating of adhesive tape is applied. Where the splint is angled, the tape may be cut and the edges overlapped to create a smooth appearance.

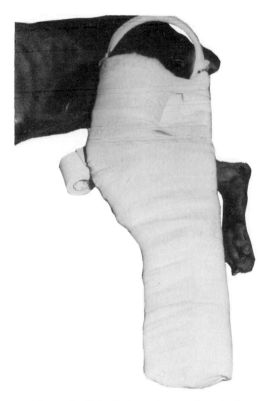

Figure 8–126 Taping is continued in as smooth a fashion as possible.

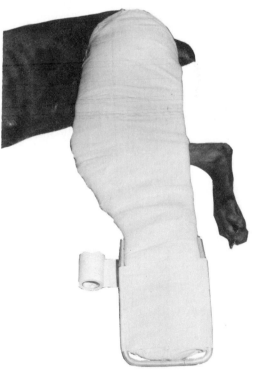

Figure 8–127 A piece of combine bandage is placed lateral to the hip, and the taping is completed; an aluminum rod stirrup is applied.

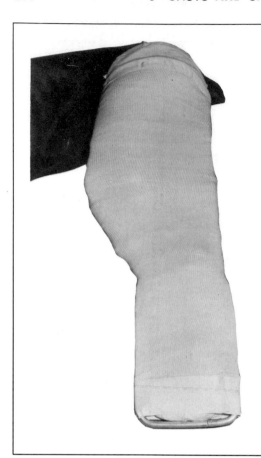

Figure 8–128 A stockinette is applied temporarily and is removed before discharge.

Forelimb Schroeder-Thomas Splint

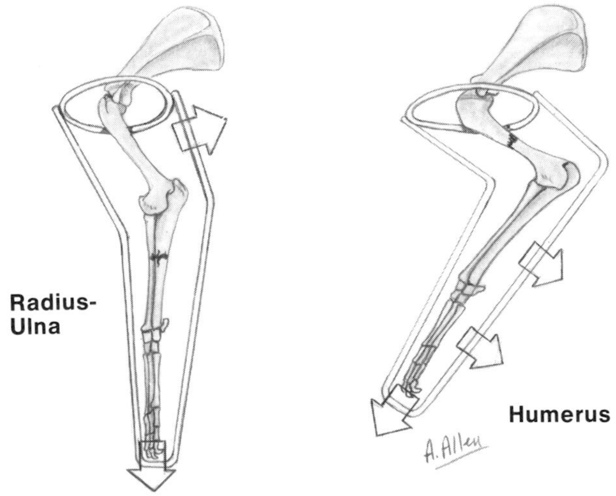

Radius-
Ulna

Humerus

A. Allen

Figure 8–129   Configurations of splints for fractures of the fore-limb.

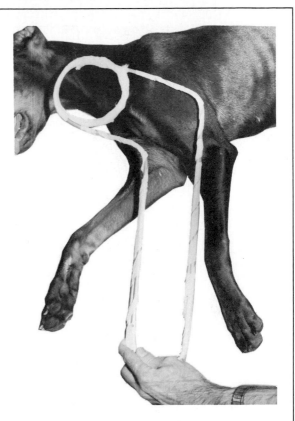

Figure 8–130 A properly structured splint for fracture of the humerus. The ring is padded and tape is applied (adhesive side out) to the splint rods.

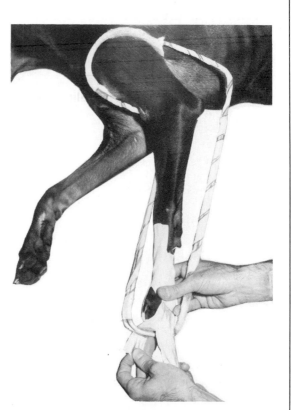

Figure 8–131 The foot is taped cranially and caudally and is rotated inward as it is fixed to the distal splint rod. Combine roll is applied from the foot proximally and is tightened.

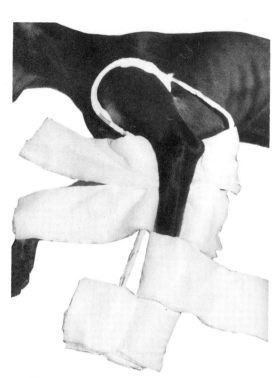

Figure 8–132 The radius and ulna are pulled caudally under marked tension with combine roll.

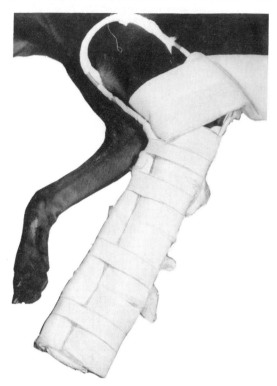

Figure 8–133 Combine bandage is more loosely applied through the region of the humerus.

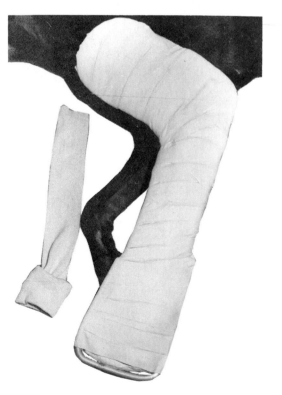

Figure 8–134 The proximal ring is closed with combine bandage and the splint is taped; an aluminum stirrup is applied to the distal end. Stockinette is applied temporarily and is removed before discharge.

FIGURE EIGHT (EHMER) SLING

The figure eight, butterfly, or Ehmer sling is designed to create flexion of the rearlimb with rotation of the femoral head into the socket. It is useful in post-reduction fixation of coxofemoral luxation in small animals. When properly applied, it may be left in place for five to seven days. The sling should be applied with the pressure maintained as evenly as possible; the proximal flank and distal foot should be examined regularly for skin inflammation and edema.

Application

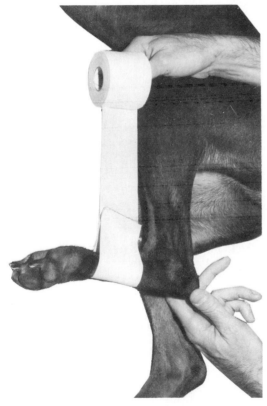

Figure 8–135 An adhesive tape sling is made for the metatarsal area.

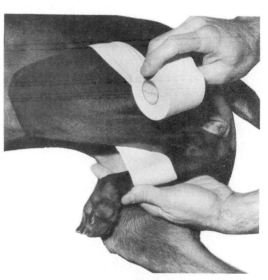

Figure 8–136 The tape is passed on the medial side of the thigh to the proximal flank and is returned to the point of origin.

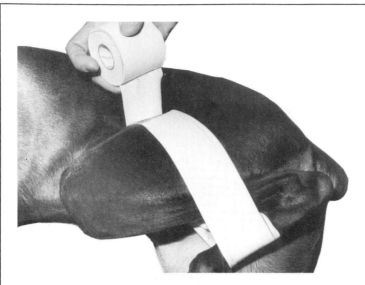

Figure 8–137 The tape is passed on the medial side of the leg to the flank again.

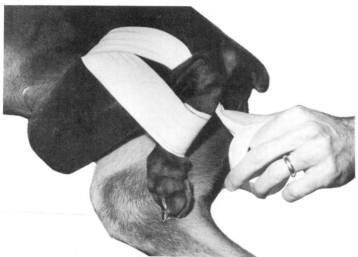

Figure 8–138 The tape is placed on the lateral thigh and medial hock.

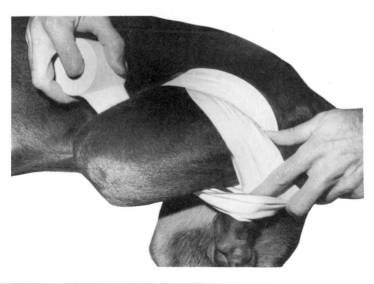

Figure 8–139 The tape is continued ventral and lateral to the metacarpal area and is again passed on the medial side of the thigh. The foot is rotated inward and the hock outward.

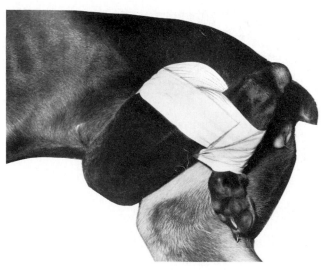

Figure 8–140 One or more layers may repeat the configuration shown in Figure 8–139.

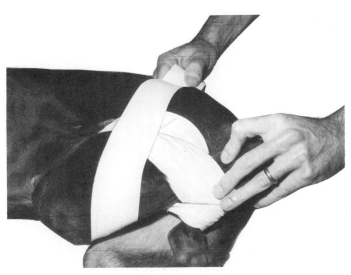

Figure 8–141 An accessory tape encircling the sling, abdomen, and back may be applied in cats and in dogs with short limbs and abundant skin in order to add additional stability to the sling.

ROBINSON SLING

A modified rearlimb sling has been devised that prevents full use of the limb with minimal flexion. It has been advocated to prevent full use following orthopedic repair of the long bones and joints. The sling is demonstrated here with minimal modifications.

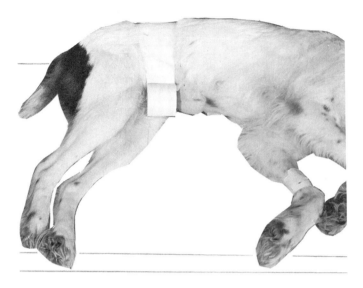

Figure 8–142 A strip of 2-inch tape is applied around the abdomen at the flank. It is applied loosely in the male.

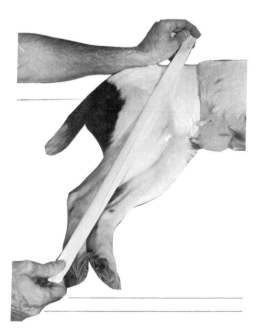

Figure 8–143 Two strips of tape are cut long enough to reach from the foot to the top of the lumbar muscles. Each is folded lengthwise with the adhesive side apposed.

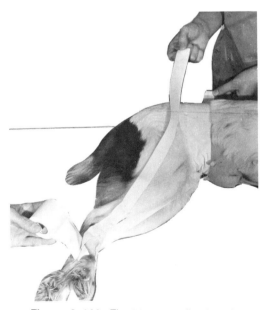

Figure 8–144 The tapes are fixed to the metatarsal area with a ring of 2-inch tape applied without pressure. One tape is passed lateral to the stifle and to the flank. The other folded tape is placed medial to the stifle and around the opposite flank.

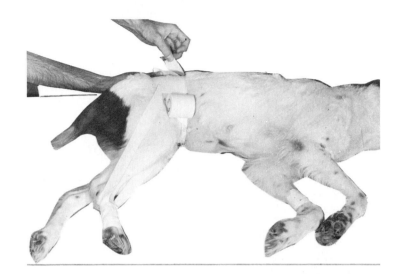

Figure 8–145 The limb is flexed beyond a normal walking position by pulling the tapes over the back. These tapes are fixed with the 2-inch tape applied over that around the abdomen.

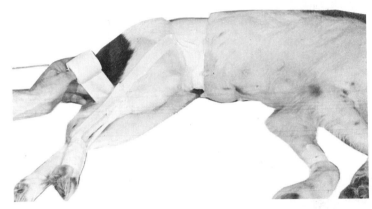

Figure 8–146 The tapes medial and lateral to the tibia are fixed with loosely applied tape. The tape need not be applied to the hair.

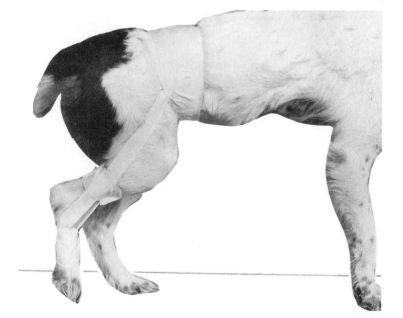

Figure 8–147 The sling allows limited extension with comfort.

SHOULDER SLING

The shoulder sling is similar to the rearlimb sling in that its primary purpose is to maintain temporary stability. The sling should be applied with a minimum of tension but must be kept firm to the skin or hair to prevent rotation and loss of stability.

Application

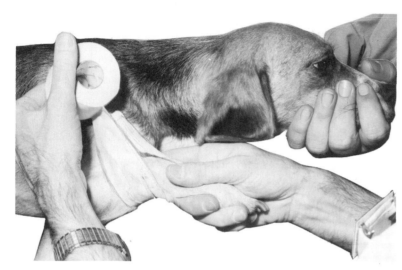

Figure 8–148 An adhesive tape stirrup is placed at the distal radial (carpal) region and is passed lateral to the brachium over the shoulders.

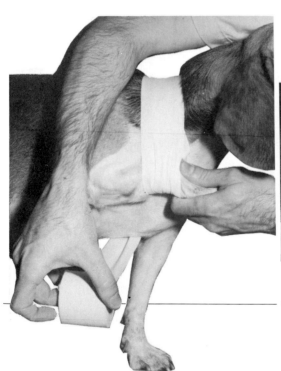

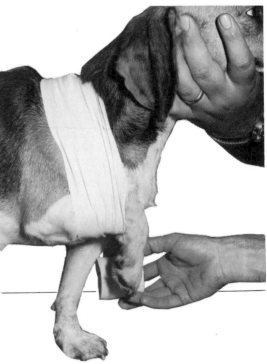

Figure 8–149 The tape is continued around the body to the point of origin.

Figure 8–150 The body and suspended limb are encircled with tape medial and lateral to the opposite limb.

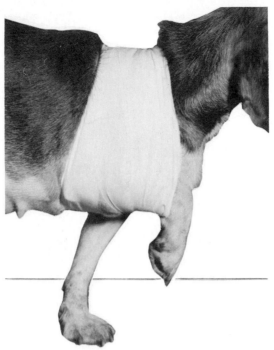

Figure 8–151 The elbow should be lower than the carpus. Particular attention should be paid to skin necrosis in the carpal region.

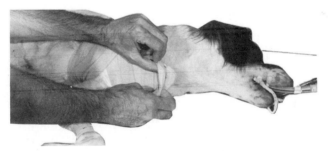

Figure 8–152 Pressure on the carpus may be prevented by turning the foot inward and extending the tape over the carpus and foot.

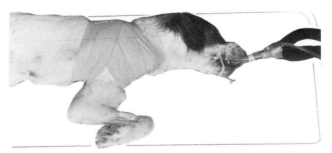

Figure 8–153 This modification of the shoulder sling is called a Velpeau bandage.

REFERENCES

Alexander, J. E., Archibald, J., and Cawley, A. J.: Pelvic fractures and their reduction in small animals. Mod. Vet. Pract., 1962, 43:9.

Anderson, R.: The Anderson splint. Surg. Gynecol. Obstet., 1936, 62:865.

Armistead, W. W., and Lumb, W. V.: Management of distal epiphyseal fractures of the femur. North Am. Vet., 1952, 33:481.

Bjorck, G.: A transfixation plaster cast in the treatment of small animals. Vet. Med., 1952, 4:89.

Brinker, W. D., and Sales, E. K.: Treatment of dislocation of the elbow in dogs. Vet. Med., 1949, 44:135.

Campbell, J. R., Lawson, D. D., and Wyburn, R. S.: Coxofemoral luxation in the dog. Vet. Rec., 1965, 77:1173.

Charnley, J.: *The Closed Treatment of Common Fractures*. Baltimore: Williams and Wilkins Co., 1957.

Cofield, R. B.: Technique in handling simple and compound fractures. North Am. Vet., 1934, 15:32.

Dammrich, K.: Pathology of growth and reconstructive processes in the cranial bones in animals (dogs and cats). Dtsch. Tierarztl Wochenschr., 1966, 73:590.

Dibbell, E. B.: Dislocation of the hip in dogs and cats. North Am. Vet., 1934, 15:37.

Dibbell, E. B.: Splints for fixation of fractures and dislocations in small animals. North Am. Vet., 1930, 11:29.

Ehmer, E. E.: Special casts for the treatment of pelvic and femoral fractures and coxofemoral luxations. N. Am. Vet., 1934, 15:31.

Frost, R. C.: The closed reduction and repair of radioulnar fractures in the dog. J. Sm. Anim. Pract., 1965, 6:197.

Hickman, J.: *Veterinary Orthopaedics*. Edinburgh: Oliver and Boyd, 1964.

Hoerlein, B. F.: Methods of spinal fusion and vertebral immobilization in the dog. Am. J. Vet. Res., 1956, 17:695.

Hohn, R. B.: Principles and application of plaster casts. Vet. Clin. North Am., 1975, 5:291.

Jennings, W. E.: Dislocation of the hip joint in the dog. Cornell Vet., 1934, 24:260.

Jenny, J.: Today's standard of fracture treatment in small animals. Proc. 89th Ann. Meet., A.V.M.A., 1953, 187:1952.

Knecht, C. D.: Application of temporary splints. Vet. Clin. North Am., 1975, 5:165.

Knecht, C. D.: Principles and application of traction and coaptation splints. Vet. Clin. North Am., 1975, 5:177.

Knowles, A. T., Knowles, J. O., and Knowles, R. P.: Clinical application of splints in fractures of the pelvis. Vet. Med., 1949, 44:308.

Leonard, E. P.: *Fundamentals of Small Animal Surgery*. Philadelphia: W. B. Saunders Co., 1968.

Leonard, E. P.: *Orthopedic Surgery of the Dog and Cat*, 2nd ed. Philadelphia, W. B. Saunders Co., 1971.

Mason, C. T.: A new appliance for metacarpal and metatarsal surgery. Auburn Vet., 1948, 4:91.

Mason, C. T.: Useful appliance for fractures of the extremities of dogs. North Am. Vet., 1948, 29:360.

McCunn, J.: Fractures and dislocations in small animals. Vet. Rec., 1933, 47:1236.

Olsen, M. L.: *Canine Surgery*, 4th ed. Evanston, Ill.; American Veterinary Publications, Inc., 1959.

Pozzi, L.: Treatment of fractures of the mandible in the dog. Atti. Soc. Ital. Sci. Vet., 1969, 14:214.

Schroeder, E. F.: Injuries in the region of the hip in small animals. J.A.V.M.A., 1936, 89:522.

Schroeder, E. F.: The traction principle in treating fractures and dislocations in the dog and cat. North Am. Vet., 1933, 14:32.

Schroeder, E. F., and Schnelle, G. B.: The stifle joint. North Am. Vet., 1941, 22:353.

Stader, O.: Dislocation of the hip joint. North Am. Vet., 1955, 36:1026.

Waterman, N. G., Stockinger, T., and Goldblatt, D.: Effects of various dressings on skin and subcutaneous temperatures. Arch. Surg., 1967, 95:464.

White, C. A.: Bilateral forward mandibular luxation in a dog. North Am. Vet., 1959, 30:777.

9

CASTS AND SPLINTS FOR LARGE ANIMALS

9

CASTS AND SPLINTS FOR LARGE ANIMALS

INTRODUCTION TO EQUINE CASTING

Casts are used to partially or completely immobilize a part. In the horse, casting may be used to cover severe wounds to allow healing, to add support to an inflamed tendon, to help treat contracted tendons in the young, and to help immobilize fractures.

Cast material and design should be selected for each case. Vet Set* can be used as a rigid support bandage or as a cast base. Plaster of Paris or resin-impregnated gauze can be used over the cast base. Stockinette and orthopedic felt or some other type of padding used at pressure points is probably the most common padding used.

A cast may be applied with or without a walking bar. The walking bar adds support and may transfer weight up the limb. One important point to remember with a horse is that it will support some weight on the affected limb. This point must be taken into consideration when applying the cast.

Recovery from anesthesia, which is frequently required for cast application, is a stressful period. This is particularly true with plaster of Paris, which at that stage has not reached its full tensile strength. A cast will usually break at the site of the fractures or at the joint proximal to the fracture. Additional reinforcements are necessary at these points. Resin-impregnated gauze overcomes some of the disadvantages of plaster in that it dries rapidly and is not as heavy.

---

*Vet Set is distributed by Veterinary Products Industries, Phoenix, Ariz.

LOWER LEG SPLINT
Polyvinyl Chloride Pipe

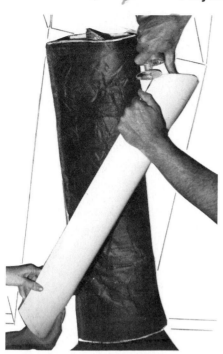

Figure 9–1 An economical splint can be constructed from polyvinyl chloride (PVC) pipe. The pipe is split lengthwise, and the edges are rounded with an oscillating cast cutter.

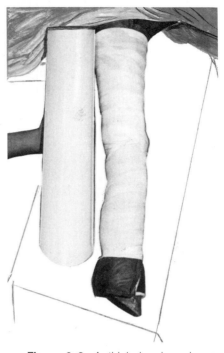

Figure 9–2 A thick bandage is applied for padding.

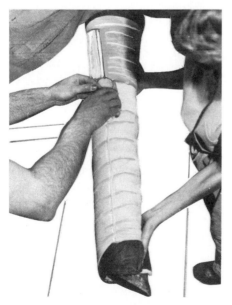

Figure 9–3 The PVC splint is held in position with elastic leg wraps.

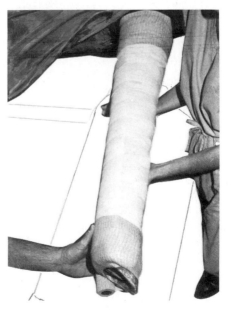

Figure 9–4 Elastic adhesive tape* may be applied to the top and bottom of the PVC splint to prevent slippage.

*Elastikon Porous Adhesive Tape is manufactured by Johnson and Johnson, New Brunswick, N.J.

FOOT AND LOWER LEG CASTS
Sole Cast

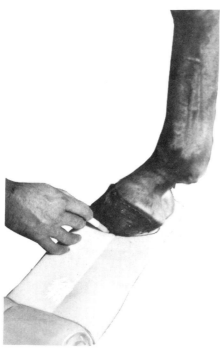

Figure 9-5 A sole cast can be made from Vet Set roll or from a roll of plaster of Paris. If Vet Set is used, the shape of the foot is outlined on the roll.

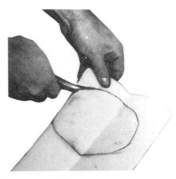

Figure 9-6 The piece should be cut slightly smaller than the outline drawing.

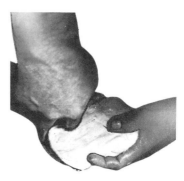

Figure 9-7 The piece is positioned and is trimmed to fit properly and to fill the sole before wetting.

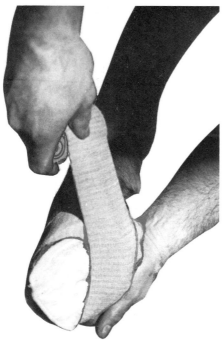

Figure 9-8 The piece of Vet Set can be held in place with plaster of Paris or elastic tape.

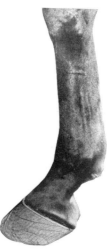

Figure 9-9 The horse is made to bear weight on a flat surface for at least 10 minutes or until the plaster hardens.

Foot Cast

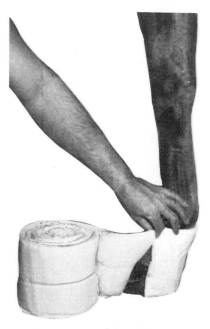

Figure 9–10 Vet Set can be applied as a conforming pressure bandage around the foot. The appropriate length of roll is measured and cut.

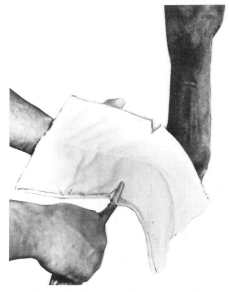

Figure 9–11 A wedge is removed on each side to help the cast conform to the foot.

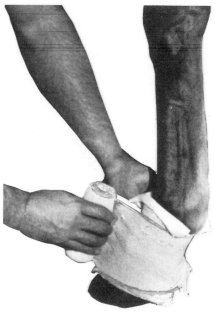

Figure 9–12 The Vet Set is wetted, wrung, and smoothed. It is wrapped snugly with elastic wrap after application.

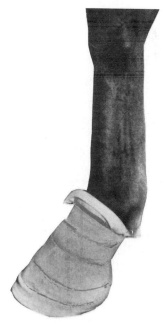

Figure 9–13 The horse is made to bear weight on the foot until the plaster begins to harden.

Fabricated Plaster Support

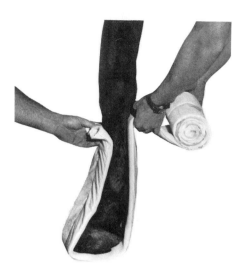

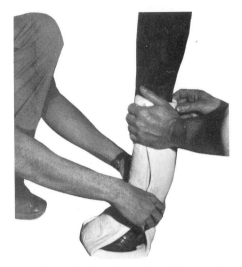

Figure 9–14   Vet Set roll can be used as a conforming bandage below the carpus or hock. A length is measured and cut.

Figure 9–15   The wet Vet Set is applied to the leg, avoiding wrinkles. The sides are overlapped, and the top is rolled outward and distally.

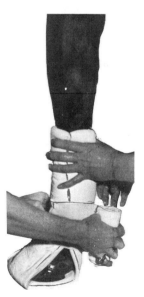

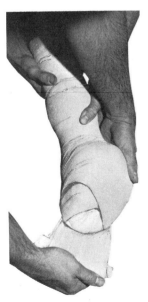

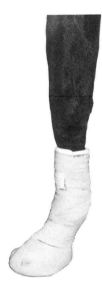

Figure 9–16   An elastic wrap is applied firmly.

Figure 9–17   The foot and cast are completely wrapped.

Figure 9–18 The horse is made to bear weight on the limb for at least 10 minutes or until the cast starts to harden.

Fabricated Plaster Removal and Reapplication

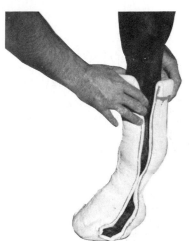

Figure 9-19 The elastic wrap is removed, and the cast is spread.

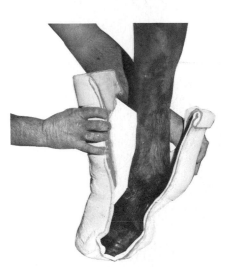

Figure 9-20 The cast can be spread enough for removal and can be replaced if desired.

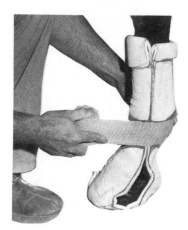

Figure 9-21 The dry cast is wrapped after reapplication. With use, the foot will wear through the cast without major problems.

Gelocast* Bandage

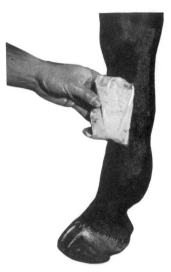

Figure 9–22 The Gelocast* is removed from the plastic outer wrap. If it is not soft and pliable it should be discarded.

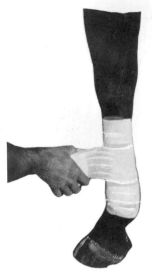

Figure 9–23 The Gelocast is wrapped smoothly and snugly on the leg.

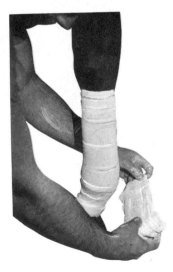

Figure 9–24 A second roll is applied and is conformed to the leg with palm pressure.

*Gelocast is manufactured by Duke Laboratories, Inc., S. Norwalk, Conn.

FULL FORELIMB CASTS
Plaster of Paris

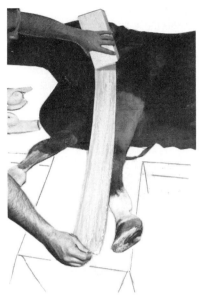

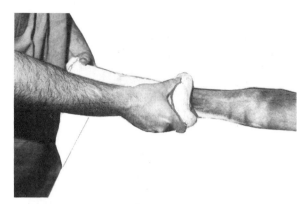

Figure 9–26 The stockinette is unrolled on the leg and then is pulled approximately one inch distally to smooth the hair.

Figure 9–25 A stockinette is measured and is cut with excess to roll at the top and bottom.

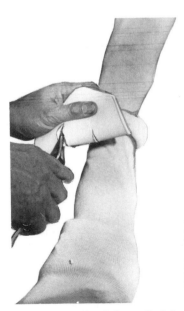

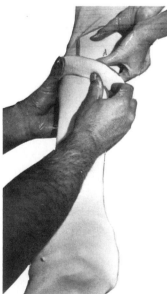

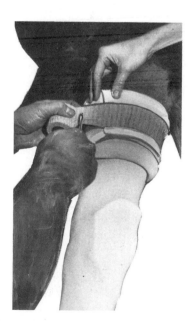

Figure 9–27 Orthopedic felt padding is cut and is applied over the accessory carpal bone and is extended around the coronary band.

Figure 9–28 The padding is covered with a second layer of stockinette.

Figure 9–29 Orthopedic felt is wrapped at the top of the proposed cast and is covered with the outer layer of stockinette.

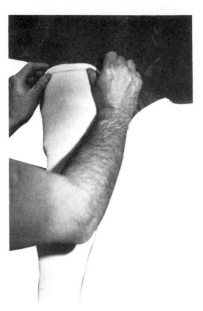

Figure 9–30 The outer stockinette is unrolled to extend above the inner wrap and felt.

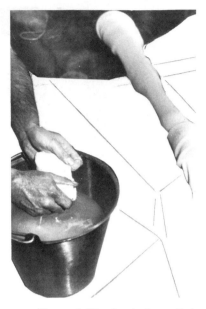

Figure 9–31 A plaster roll is saturated with water and is wrung to remove the excess.

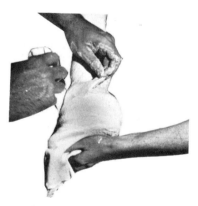

Figure 9–32 Application of the plaster is begun above the coronary band before the leg is wrapped.

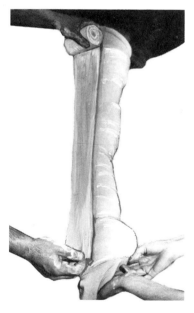

Figure 9–33 Strength without additional layers is provided by a layered longitudinal plaster strip. The length is measured, and an entire roll of plaster is overlapped to make the support.

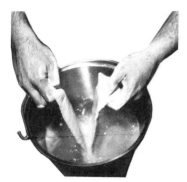

Figure 9–34 The layered plaster strip is immersed in warm water and is wrung.

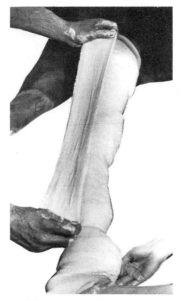

Figure 9–35 The plaster strip is applied to the leg.

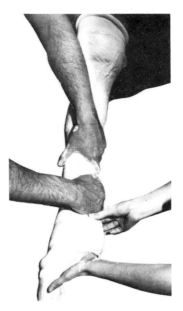

Figure 9–36 The plaster is conformed to the leg with palm pressure.

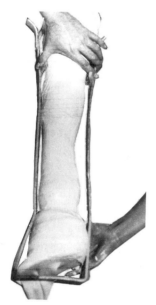

Figure 9–37 A reinforcing bar can be applied in a cranial to caudal direction or in a medial to lateral direction to add strength.

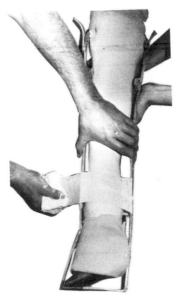

Figure 9–38 The reinforcing bar is fixed.

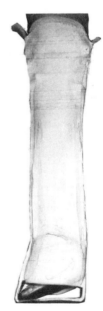

Figure 9–39 In the completed cast, the foot is exposed and the top is wrapped loosely with elastic tape to prevent the entrance of bedding between the cast and the leg.

Removing the Plaster Cast

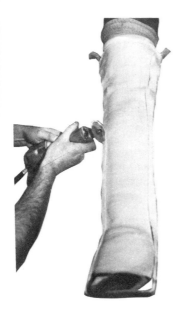

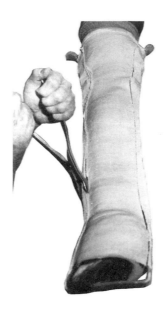

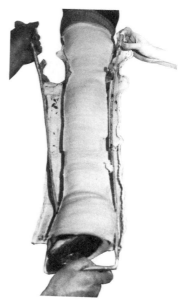

Figure 9–40 An oscillating cast-cutting saw is used to score the full length of the cast parallel to the walking bar on each side.

Figure 9–41 A cast spreader is used to separate the layers of plaster that hold the walking bar.

Figure 9–42 The walking bar is spread slightly and is removed.

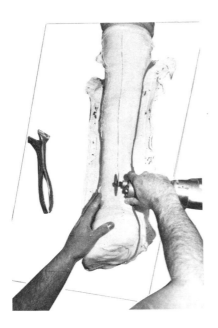

Figure 9–43 The oscillating saw is used carefully to cut through the cast. The saw should not be pulled as it cuts through the cast. It should be pressed inward with controlled motion. As soon as the blade goes through the plaster, it is withdrawn, moved slightly, and pressed again. The thumb is used as a depth gauge to prevent excess penetration because the underlying skin is not as pliable as normal skin and is easily cut with the blade.

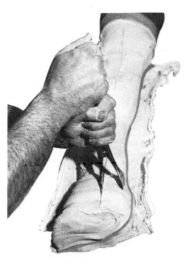

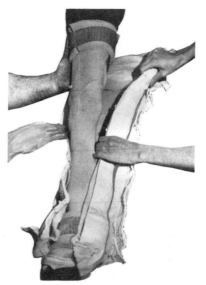

Figure 9–44 One blade of a cast spreader is placed in the saw track and is rotated to spread the cast sufficiently for introduction of both blades. A cut may be made on the opposite side of the cast to help separation.

Figure 9–45 Traction is needed on both sides of the cast to remove it from the leg.

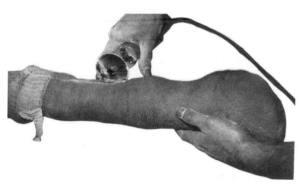

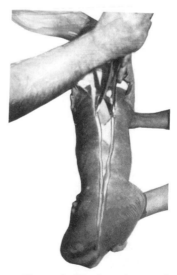

Figure 9–46 Casts applied with other substances, such as the resin-impregnated material shown, are removed by the same procedures. The thumb is again used as a depth gauge. The saw blade will become hot during removal of this cast.

Figure 9–47 A cast spreader is used. A second cut may be necessary to remove the cast from the leg.

Fabricated Plaster* and Resin-Impregnated Gauze†‡
Application

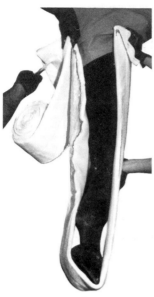

Figure 9–48 Vet Set is a layered plaster stitched between a layer of cloth on one side and foam on the other. The measured length is sufficient to permit a fold at the top.

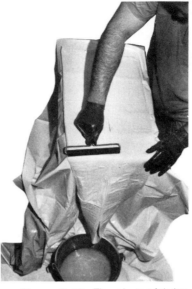

Figure 9–49 The plaster fabrication is thoroughly wet and vigorously wrung. A roller is used to smooth and help bond the layers.

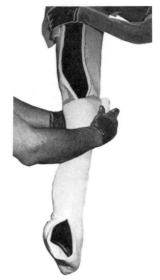

Figure 9–50 The Vet Set is applied to the leg and is wrapped with elastic bandage, which is removed after the plaster hardens in approximately 10 minutes.

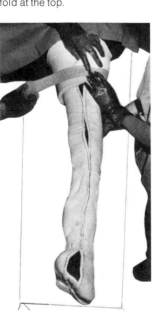

Figure 9–51 A wide piece of felt is measured and is applied around the limb at the top of the cast.

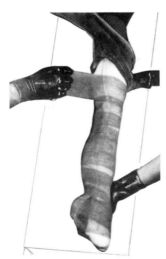

Figure 9–52 Resin-impregnated gauze is applied over the Vet Set. Disposable gloves should be worn during application.

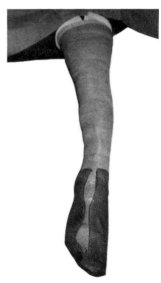

Figure 9–53 A splint of resin-impregnated gauze is applied over the foot and is held in place with similar roll material.

*Vet Set is distributed by Veterinary Products Industries, Phoenix, Ariz.
†Cutter Cast Tape is available from Cutter Biomedical, San Diego, Ca.
‡Hexcelite Orthopaedic Tape is manufactured by Hexcel Medical Products, Dublin, Ca.

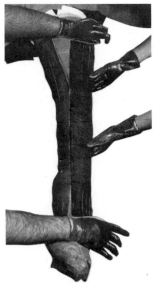

Figure 9–54 A similar splint is applied to the cranial and caudal surfaces to add strength with minimal weight.

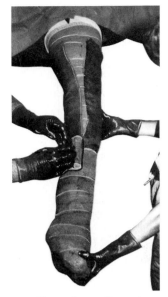

Figure 9–55 The splints are fixed with resin-impregnated gauze.

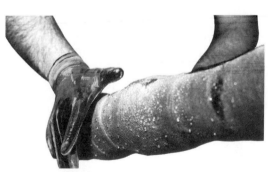

Figure 9–56 The cast is smoothed and bubbles are removed with a rolling motion of the palms of the hands.

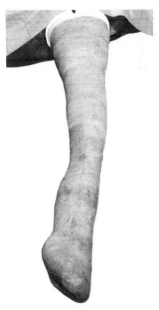

Figure 9–57 The finished cast is lightweight and strong.

Cast Removal

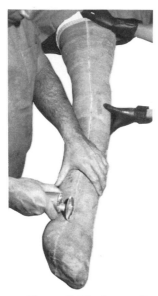 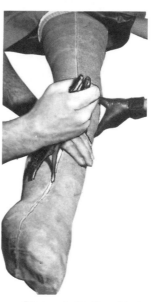 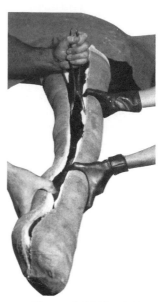

Figure 9–58 An oscillating saw is used carefully to cut each side of the cast and to cut around the foot (Fig. 9–43).

Figure 9–59 One blade of a cast spreader is inserted in the slot and is twisted to separate the cast enough for both blades.

Figure 9–60 The halves of the cast are separated and removed.

Cast Reapplication

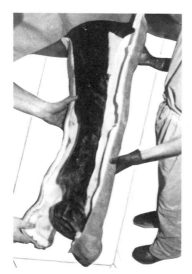 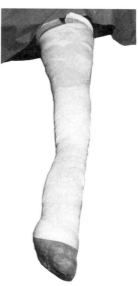

Figure 9–61 The halves can be reapplied to the leg for recovery from anesthesia or to extend immobilization.

Figure 9–62 The cast is wrapped with elastic tape. The end of the cast can be removed for weight-bearing on the foot.

REARLIMB CASTS

Resin-Impregnated

Application

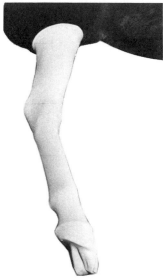

Figure 9–63 A stockinette is measured, cut, and unrolled on the leg.

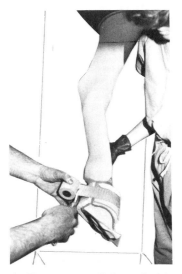

Figure 9–64 Orthopedic felt is cut and is fixed around the coronet with adhesive tape.

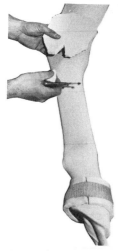

Figure 9–65 Orthopedic felt is cut to fit over the point of the hock. The felt is notched at the bottom and top to prevent wrinkles.

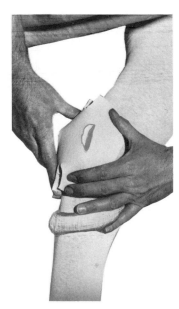

Figure 9–66 The felt is also cut on each side of the point of the hock, and a second layer of stockinette is applied over the felt and first layer of stockinette.

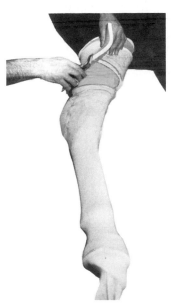

Figure 9–67 A wide piece of felt is measured and is cut to fit around the limb at the top of the cast.

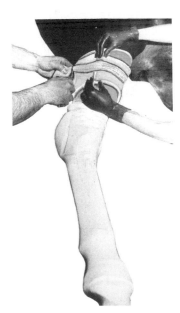

Figure 9–68 The felt is fixed with tape and then is covered with the second layer of stockinette.

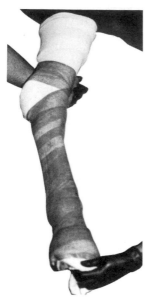

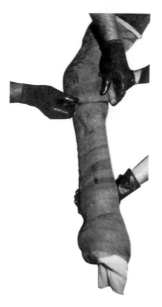

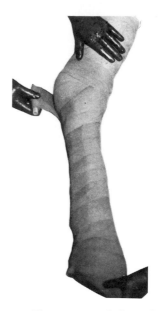

Figure 9–69 Resin-impregnated gauze is applied smoothly, starting from the foot. Disposable gloves should be worn.

Figure 9–70 The gauze casting material is folded to conform to the hock.

Figure 9–71 A figure-8 application around the hock adds additional strength.

Removal of the Cast

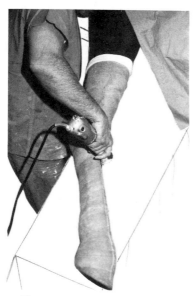

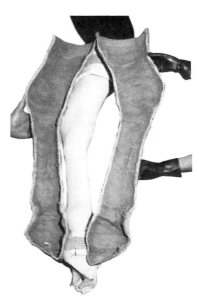

Figure 9–72 An oscillating saw is used to cut the front and rear of the cast.

Figure 9–73 The halves are separated and removed.

Fabricated Plaster and Resin-Impregnated Gauze

Application

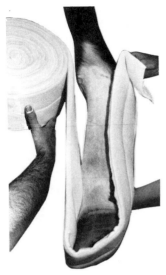

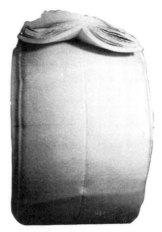

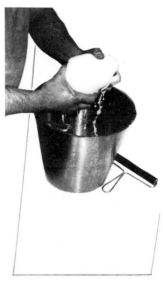

Figure 9–74 Vet Set is measured to the proper length and is cut.

Figure 9–75 The fabricated cast material consists of 15 layers of plaster with a cotton backing on one side and a layer of foam on the skin side.

Figure 9–76 The length of Vet Set is saturated with warm water and is vigorously wrung.

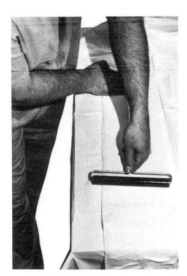

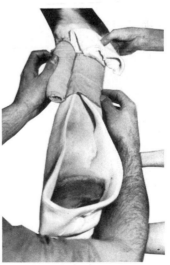

Figure 9–77 A roller is used on the cotton side to remove excess water and wrinkles and to bind the laminations.

Figure 9–78 The fabricated plaster is placed on the leg and is wrapped with an elastic wrap. The elastic wrap is removed in approximately 10 minutes when the plaster hardens.

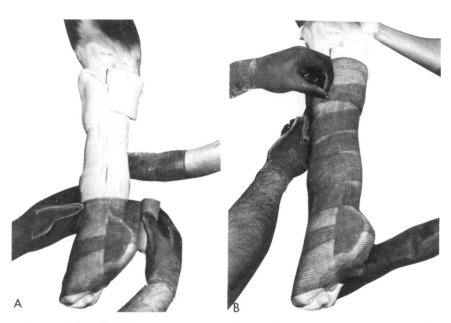

Figure 9–79 Resin-impregnated gauze is applied over the base made by the Vet Set.

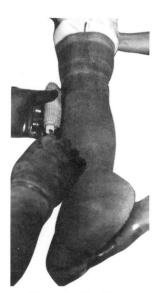

Figure 9–80 The entire foot and leg are wrapped.

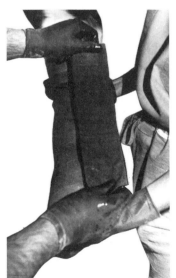

Figure 9–81 A strip of resin-impregnated gauze is conformed to the cast to add strength with minimal weight.

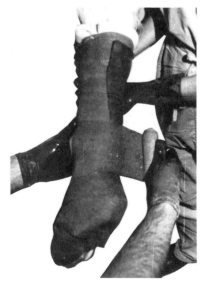

Figure 9–82 A final roll of resin-impregnated gauze is used to incorporate the reinforcing strip into the cast.

10

CARDIOPULMONARY RESUSCITATION

10

CARDIOPULMONARY RESUSCITATION

Cardiopulmonary arrest is the sudden cessation of respiration and effective circulation. Respiratory arrest may precede and contribute to cardiac arrest, or they may occur simultaneously. Cardiopulmonary arrest may result from primary cardiac or pulmonary disease, pneumothorax, pleural effusion, anemia, shock, acid-base or electrolyte imbalance, head trauma, vagal stimulation, or toxemia. It may also result iatrogenically from preanesthetic and anesthetic agents, inadequate tissue oxygenation (for example, from airway obstruction from a foreign body or a kinked endotracheal tube), patient positioning that decreases pulmonary excursion, or surgical manipulation during cardiac catheterization or surgery.

Most iatrogenic factors can be avoided or controlled. The clinician must be aware of factors that can contribute to arrest, must avoid those that are definitely contributory, and must weigh the potential benefit and harm of those that cannot be avoided.

CLINICAL SIGNS

The clinical signs of impending cardiopulmonary arrest include weak or irregular pulse, progressive arrhythmia, increased capillary refill time, alterations in respiratory pattern, particularly increased rate and decreased volume, and cyanosis. Cyanosis of the mucous membranes or capillary blood is usually a late sign and indicates profound hypoxia.

The signs of definitive arrest include apnea or apneustic gasps, absence of pulse or heart beat, dilated pupils, lack of bleeding from cut surfaces, and unconsciousness (if the patient is not anesthetized). Electrocardiographic signs are used to verify arrhythmias or cardiac arrest.

MANAGEMENT

Each hospital should have a totally equipped emergency kit or "crash cart." Stocks of drugs and supplies should be used only for emergencies and should be replaced as soon as possible after use. The contents of a standard emergency cart are listed in Table 10–1.

Several schemes have been published for the management of cardiopulmonary arrest. The primary scheme proposed here is reprinted with the permission of the American Animal Hospital Association and Dr. Walter E. Weirich. Some modifications as proposed by others are noted where they appear (Table 10–2).

Actions at the time of arrest or impending arrest should be nearly reflex. For this reason, an A. B. C. approach is recommended. In each instance the first step is a rapid evaluation of the state of the patient. The evaluation should include ventilatory motion, palpation for heart beat and femoral pulse, evaluation of color and capillary refill of mucous membranes, and pupil size and response to light. As soon as arrest has been validated, the attendant should do the following:

A — Establish a patent AIRWAY
B — BREATHE for the patient
C — Restore the CIRCULATION
D — Give DRUGS and/or DEFIBRILLATE
E — EVALUATE the clinical and electrocardiographic status of the patient

TABLE 10–1   Standard Emergency Kit

Standard Emergency Kit	Emergency Surgery Tray (Sterile)	Equipment	Drugs
Oxygen source	Scalpel and blade	ECG monitor	Heparinized saline
Lighted laryngoscope	Hemostats	Esophageal stethoscope	Infusion solutions
Assorted endotracheal tubes	Thumb forceps	Audio-patient monitor	0.9% saline
Anesthetic machine or Ambu-bag	Scissors (Metzenbaum)		5% dextrose in water
Gauze and adhesive tape	Needle holders	Optional:	Lactated Ringer's solution
Indwelling catheters, 18 and 21 gauge	Rib retractor (Finochietto)	Electrical defibrillator	Atropine sulfate
Butterfly administrative needles	Sterile gloves		Calcium gluceptate (20%)
Tourniquet	Sterile sponges		or gluconate (10%)
Alcohol wipes	Suture materials		Dexamethasone
Intravenous infusion sets			Diazepam
Needles—20, 18, and 16 gauge			Digoxin
Syringes			Doxapram
1 cc.			Epinephrine (1:1,000, 1:10,000)
3 cc.			Isoproterenol HCl
6 cc. } multiples should			Levallorphan tartrate
12 cc. } be available			Lidocaine without epinephrine (2%)
20 cc.			Mannitol (20%)
35 cc.			Sodium bicarbonate
			Sterile water for injection

A—Airway

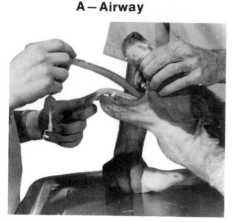

Figure 10–1   An endotracheal tube is placed.

B—Breathe

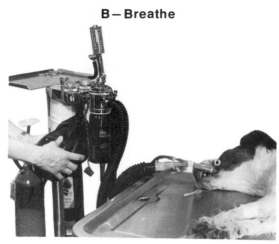

Figure 10–2   Ventilation is initiated.

An endotracheal tube is placed and the cuff is inflated. A lighted laryngoscope should be available for those wishing to use it. Should intubation not be possible, a tracheostomy should be performed.

Ventilation is initiated with 100 per cent oxygen through an anesthetic machine or Ambu-bag (Table 10–2a). A pressure-limited ventilator should not be used because pressure on the chest during cardiac

TABLE 10–2   Treatment of Cardiopulmonary Arrest

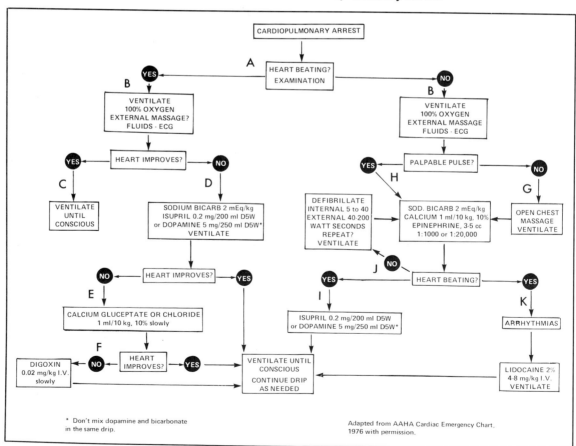

* Don't mix dopamine and bicarbonate in the same drip.

Adapted from AAHA Cardiac Emergency Chart, 1976 with permission.

massage will interrupt the respiratory phase. Approximately 12 to 16 breaths per minute should be given.

The heart and arterial pulse should be palpated. If a weak pulse is felt, ventilation is continued and circulatory support is given. If no pulse is evident, closed chest cardiac massage is begun.

C—Restore Circulation

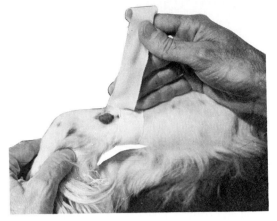

Figure 10–4 An intravenous line is established through an indwelling catheter.

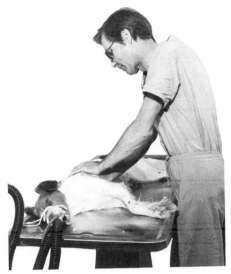

Figure 10–3 Closed cardiac massage.

Closed cardiac massage is performed with the animal in lateral recumbency with its feet towards the clinician. In small animals the palms may be compressed from each side of the chest. In larger dogs, one palm is placed over the heart, the other hand is placed on the first hand, and the fingers are locked to prevent finger pressure. Massage should compress the chest 20 to 30 per cent or enough to cause a palpable femoral pulse. The clinician should stand over the animal and should compress vertically 60 to 80 times per minute. The hand should not be lifted from the animal between compressions to reduce a "beating" effect.

If unassisted, the clinician should perform 15 compressions and stop for two rapid ventilations. When assisted, the bag should be inflated as the clinician completes each fifth massage. No delay or discontinuation of massage should be needed if one of those present counts massages aloud.

Expansion of blood volume with isotonic fluids should be begun as soon as possible. An intravenous line is established through an indwelling catheter. Lactated Ringer's solution is the solution most commonly administered. The rate should be sufficient to restore a palpable pulse on closed cardiac massage but should be controlled to prevent pulmonary edema in cats and small dogs. *The clinician who recognizes that anesthesia and surgery may incite arrest recognizes that an indwelling intravenous catheter should be placed in every animal subjected to surgery, whethert routine or complicated.*

An electrocardiogram should be obtained as soon as possible (Table 10–2B). Each employee should know how to operate the ECG monitor or strip recorder.

D—Give Drugs
and
E—Evaluate

A difference of opinion exists regarding the timing and use of specific drugs. If spontaneous heart beat and arterial pulse return, cardiac massage, but not ventilation, may be discontinued (Table 10–2C). If the pulse quality and rate continue to improve ventilation is continued until the animal is awake or breathing spontaneously. Required surgery may be rapidly completed. Elective procedures should be delayed until a later date. Treatment for cerebral edema with adrenocorticosteroids and mannitol may be required following even brief cardiopulmonary arrest.

If the quality of the pulse does not improve, the animal should be given sodium bicarbonate 2 mEq per kg. (1 mEq per lb.) intravenously, followed by isoproterenol HCl (Isuprel) at 0.2 mg. per 200 ml. D5W IV drip (Table 10–2D). An alternative to Isuprel is dopamine HCl (Intropin) 5 mg. to 250 ml. D5W. Each is given slowly to effect. Drugs should be given and ventilation should be continued until the animal is conscious.

If the heart rate and pulse quality do not improve, two drugs may be given in sequence. Calcium gluceptate (1 ml. per 10 kg.) or calcium chloride (0.05 to 0.10 cc. per kg.) should be given slowly intravenously (Table 10–2E). *Rapid injection may cause asystole.* If no response occurs, digoxin (Lanoxin) is given at 0.02 mg. per kg. IV slowly (Table 10–2F).

The effectiveness of cardiac massage will alter the course of therapy. If a palpable pulse is not achieved by closed chest massage, the thorax should be opened at the left fifth intercostal space (Table 10–2G). Long hair may be rapidly clipped or parted. Short hair is not clipped. Alcohol wipes are used to spread the hair, and the skin and intercostal muscles and pleura are incised. A rib spreader is inserted, and the pericardial sac is incised. Effective internal massage is improved by wide incision of the pericardium, but the phrenic nerve should not be severed. The heart is cupped in the palm of one hand and is compressed. The descending aorta may be compressed against the vertebral column to increase coronary and cerebral perfusion.

If resuscitation is successful, the heart is observed for five minutes. The thorax is lavaged with Ringer's solution or saline and is routinely closed. A drain tube may be placed through an adjacent intercostal space and attached to a Heimlich valve.

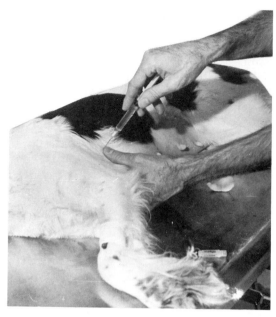

Figure 10-5 Intracardiac injection.

is given by intravenous or intracardiac injection, and massage and ventilation are continued. Finally, 3 to 5 cc. of epinephrine is given. Some prefer dilution to 1:10,000; the author gives 1:1000 solution (1 to 2 cc.).

Intracardiac injection is frequently the route of choice for these drugs. The premeasured dose is injected via a 1 to 1½ in. 20 to 21 gauge needle. If the chest is open, the drug in injected into the left ventricle, and the heart is massaged as the descending aorta is compressed. If the chest is closed, the heart is palpated at the fifth intercostal space at a point immediately caudal to the point of the elbow and slightly dorsal to the costochondral junction. The skin, intercostal space, and ventricle are penetrated, the syringe is aspirated to reveal blood, and the drug is injected as a bolus.

ASYSTOLE

If the heart does not begin beating but a palpable pulse is achieved with closed or open chest massage, a sequence of drugs is given (Table 10–2H). Sodium bicarbonate is given first at 2 mEq per kg. by intravenous or intracardiac injection. Massage and ventilation are continued. If spontaneous heart beat does not occur, 1 ml. per 10 kg. 10 per cent calcium gluceptate or calcium chloride

SPONTANEOUS PULSE

Spontaneous pulse should begin. If not, the drugs are repeated in the same order, and massage and ventilation are continued. If spontaneous heart beat occurs, the quality and rate of pulse are monitored. If necessary, isoproterenol (0.2 mg. per 200 ml. D5W) or dopamine (5 mg. to 250 ml. D5W) is given by slow drip to effect (Table 10–2I).

If spontaneous but ineffective heart action returns, ventricular fibrillation or flutter should be suspected. The electrocardiogram should be examined to confirm these findings, and defibrillation should be attempted (Table 10–2J).

Defibrillation is best performed with an electric defibrillator. The paddles should be covered with saline-soaked sponges and should be applied directly to each side of the heart in the open-chested dog or with paste on each side of the thorax if the chest is closed. Initial defibrillation should be attempted with low power (5 to 40 watt-seconds at 1 watt-second per kg.) internally. External application will require higher power (40 to 200 watt-seconds depending on body weight) in two to three short, repetitive bursts. The clinician should hold the paddles properly and should remove all paste from his hands. All personnel should be away from the table and ventilation bag before defibrillation. Drug (sodium bicarbonate, calcium, epinephrine) and electrical defibrillation should be alternated if response does not occur.

Chemical defibrillation is more difficult. A mixture of potassium chloride and acetylcholine has been recommended. The dose is 1 mEq KCl plus 5 mg. acetylcholine per kg. body weight. It is not recommended unless an electrical defibrillator is not available.

ARRHYTHMIAS

Cardiac arrhythmias may be observed during respiratory arrest or following injection of emergency drugs. Lidocaine may be given in 2 per cent solution (4 to 8 mg. per kg.) IV to suppress arrhythmias (Table 10–2K).

The signs of successful resuscitation are return of spontaneous heart beat and pulses, bleeding from cut surfaces, improved color of mucous membranes, shortening of capillary refill time, miosis, and voluntary respiration. Electroencephalographic evidence of brain function is a valuable adjunct but rarely is available. Cerebral edema may be presumed and should be treated with corticosteroids and intravenous mannitol. Pulmonary edema as a result of excess fluid loading and hypoxia may be treated with corticosteroids, diuretics, and positive end expiratory pressure ventilation. Discrepancies in blood gases should be corrected based on sequential analysis.

Cardiopulmonary arrests will occur in spite of good medical and surgical care. Successful resuscitation requires team effort. The best time to practice is when no real emergency exists. No reading can replace the reflex responses learned during mock arrests.

REFERENCES

A.A.H.A. Cardiology Committee: The A.A.H.A. emergency chart. American Animal Hospital Association, 1976.

Bonagura, J.: Cardiovascular emergencies. Proceedings of 6th American Animal Hospital Association meeting, 1979, 49–55.

INDEX

Numbers in *italics* refer to page numbers of illustrations; numbers followed by (t) refer to tables.

Cardiac Emergency Chart

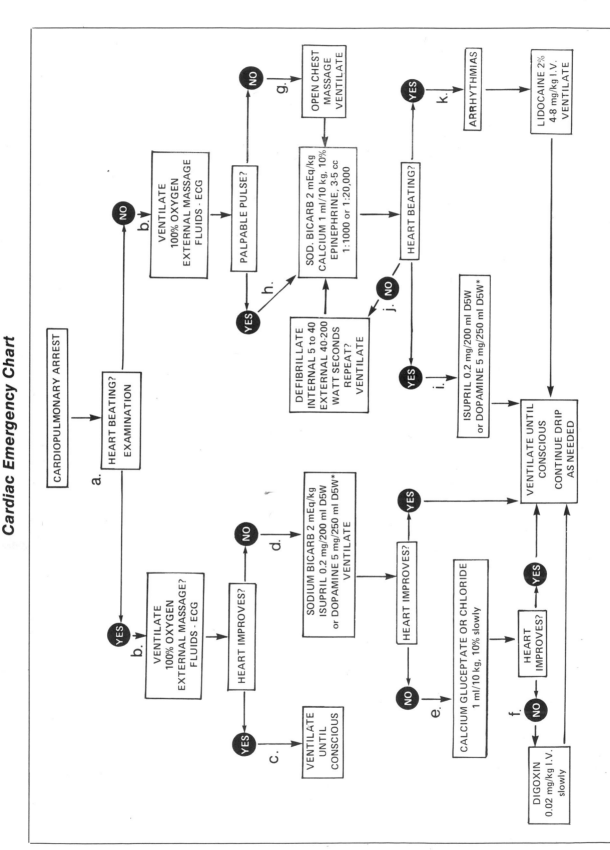

Adapted from AAHA Cardiac Emergency Chart

* Don't mix dopamine and bicarbonate